Praise for NEURO—

"Instructive . . . authoritative."

Publishers Weekly

"An impressive array of topics and much engrossing detail."

Library Journal

"Compelling . . . Engrossing medical journalism . . . What Noonan states with authority, he also states with brilliance."

Booklist

"Acutely observed . . . Noonan explores not only the 'miracles' of neurology, but also its sins."

The Kirkus Reviews

NEURO:

*Life on the Frontlines
of Brain Surgery
and Neurological Medicine*

David Noonan

IVY BOOKS · NEW YORK

Ivy Books
Published by Ballantine Books
Copyright © 1989 by David Noonan

Library of Congress Catalog Card Number: 88-36812

ISBN 0-8041-0598-7

This edition published by arrangement with Simon and Schu-
ster, Inc.

*Material in Chapter VIII is quoted from Walter Freeman and
James W. Watts*, Psychosurgery in the Treatment of Mental
Disorders and Intractable Pain, *2nd Edition, 1950. Courtesy of
Charles C. Thomas, Publisher, Springfield, Illinois.*

Manufactured in the United States of America

First Ballantine Books Edition: April 1990

For Susan

CONTENTS

What is a man anyhow? What am I? and what are you?

—WALT WHITMAN
Leaves of Grass

PREFACE

THERE is nothing in nature as perfect or as powerful as the human nervous system—not the seamless folding of the seasons one into the other; not the rolling, biogenetic mass of the oceans; not the great silent spin of the planets around the sun. The nervous system fires every human act, drives every human moment. It enables man to think and to move, to feel and to wonder, and makes him the dominant life form in the known universe. A charged web that hangs in every human body, its electrochemical circuits carry the elusive spark of life itself. And if that which is human is also somehow divine, then nervous tissue is both the means of the miracle and the miracle itself. Complex beyond man's understanding, the human nervous system is the most sophisticated arrangement of cells that exists.

William Shakespeare at his desk, Albert Einstein at his blackboard, Brooks Robinson at third base, Pablo Casals in concert, Henri Matisse at his easel. These are examples of the human nervous system at work. The composition of *Hamlet*, the formulation of the theory of relativity, the flawless fielding of a line drive, and the rendering of order and beauty in music and painting are all products of the nervous system. Neurons fire in unknown patterns and the world is seen, the universe is understood, man's nature is explored, the ball game is saved.

1

So many and so varied are the functions of the nervous system it seems incredible that they can all be traced back to the same anatomy, that the honed reflexes of a Hall of Fame baseball player and the conceptual powers of a scientific genius could originate in the same place. But the nervous system does it all. It is responsible for everything, from the purely physical to the purely cerebral, from the fact of a beating heart to the fantasy of a dream.

The enormous complexity of the nervous system engages microbiologists, psychiatrists, biochemists, philosophers, cognitive scientists, and many more medical and scientific types, each trying to get a grip on his own particular piece of the thing. As never before, the push is on to understand how the nervous system does what it does. Some scientists are trying to figure out the basic chemistry of the nervous system; they want to identify the chemical composition of the scores of neurotransmitters that link the millions of nerve cells that make up an individual nervous system. Others are interested in the ancient matter of the ''mind.'' What is it? How does it work? Where and how does it arise in the physical stuff of blood and tissue? Still others are looking into the mysteries of specific functions, such as memory.

But of all the people working on the nervous system, the doctors involved in the routine practice of neurological medicine experience it in its most complete and intense form—whole, embedded in human beings. Neurologists and neurosurgeons are in daily contact with the entire system, and the wonder of their work is the wonder of the thing itself.

This book is about the practice of neurological medicine—the everyday business of confronting the extraordinary. It is about neurologists, neurosurgeons, and their patients, and the disorders of the nervous system that they face together. It is about cutting open human heads and cutting into the human brain. It is about mysterious diseases that disrupt and destroy man's most fundamental physical and mental faculties, and about the efforts to overcome them. And by extension it is about the human nervous system itself, because the awesome beauty of a healthy nervous system is never clearer or more palpable than when considered in the fractured light of an unhealthy one.

To approach an understanding of what the nervous system is, what it does, and how it works, you can begin by thinking of it as a kind of membrane. There is a two-way flow of energy through the membrane. On one side is the individual human being, and on the other side, the rest of the world—lovers, accidents, weather, families, meals, beaches, strangers, work, play, beer, the whole deal. Everything that is on the outside gets to the individual through his nervous system; all the various stimuli pass through it. Likewise, the individual gets to the outside world by way of his nervous system; his words and actions pass through it and affect things on the outside. Man is aware of the world outside himself because his nervous system receives and processes all the information that enables him to conclude that the world exists. And man is able to interact with that world because his nervous system provides him with the means to do so.

This makes the nervous system sound like a fancy radio, sending and receiving information, and it is, but of course there's more to it than that. The nervous system *is* the man. It's his mind—generating thought and emotion—and it's his body—monitoring and regulating the most vital functions. Without exaggeration, the human body can be seen as an elaborate machine occupied and operated by the nervous system for the primary purpose of keeping the nervous system alive and moving about. Without it, the body is nothing more than a skin bag filled with bones and exotic meats.

The thing that makes the nervous system so interesting—its ubiquity in the body—is what makes neurological medicine so tough. A bad kidney is a bad kidney, a bad lung is a bad lung. But a bad nervous system can manifest as just about anything. Like the functions of the nervous system, neurological disorders range from the mundane to the remarkable and baffling. Lower back pain can be a neurological problem and so can blindness. Alzheimer's disease, in which the cerebral cortex seems simply to rot away, is a neurological disorder, and so is carpal tunnel syndrome, in which the median nerve is compressed at the wrist and movement of the hand becomes restricted and painful. Memory loss can mean the onset of serious neurological disease and so can a twitching muscle in the forearm. When patients show up complaining of headaches or seizures or numbness or "feeling strange, not myself," or even unconscious, the neurologist or neurosurgeon has to review the wiring, trace the circuitry, and pinpoint the problem as quickly as possible. He has to know the anatomy.

There are certain courses in the medical school curriculum that serve a mean but critical role in the creation of new doctors—they drive most of the people who take them absolutely crazy while convincing a very few that they have, at last, found their calling. Neuroanatomy is one such course, as anyone who has taken it will testify. Without question one of the most difficult subjects a medical student must study, neuroanatomy is a bottomless sea of detail where bright young doctors-to-be, their legs encumbered by their baggy white pants, their arms filled with outsized, overweight texts, sink from sight, their fates sealed in the flat gaze of the anatomy professor. For the majority, neuroanatomy is a horror of memorization, a nightmare of charts and lists to be endured and conquered. But for the few, neuroanatomy is an awakening, an epiphany. They see the order, the logic, it makes sense to them, and they like that. So they become neurologists and neurosurgeons and they spend their careers confronting the disorder, illogic, and senselessness of neurological disease. (Irony is a dime a dozen in medicine.)

To give you an idea of the complexity of neuroanatomy, what follows is a list of the nerves in the right foot, as taken from the standard medical chart of the nervous system. From the ankle to the toes, it reads: saphenous nerve, deep peroneal nerve, superficial peroneus nerve, tibial nerve, lateral calcaneal branches, lateral dorsal cutaneous nerve, intermediate dorsal cutaneous nerve, medial dorsal cutaneous nerve, muscular branch, lateral plantar nerve, medial plantar nerve, superficial branch and deep branch of the lateral plantar nerve, common digital nerves, proper digital nerve, digital dorsal halluces-lateral & digital secundi medial nerves, dorsal digital nerves. Those last, the dorsal digital nerves, are the nerves in the four small toes.

The human nervous system is made up of three major sub-systems. There are the central nervous system, the peripheral nervous system, and the autonomic nervous system. The central nervous system consists of the brain and the spinal cord. The peripheral nervous system is composed of the many nerves that branch out from the central nervous system to the head, the trunk, the arms, and the legs. The peripheral nerves carry sensory information to the brain and they carry motor impulses from the brain to the voluntary muscles. The autonomic nervous system, probably the least familiar to the layman, is involved in the maintenance of the vital, involuntary functions like heartbeat and respiration.

First, the brain. Mysterious and intimidating to contemplate, the human brain is the most complex thing there is and the most difficult task it can undertake is to understand itself. The brain can be divided into two basic parts—the brainstem and the cerebral cortex. The brainstem is the core of the brain and the oldest part of the brain, in evolutionary terms. Located in the lower center of the brain, and in an adult about the size of a one-year-old's fist, it connects the brain to the spinal cord and, hence, to the rest of the nervous system. The brainstem keeps you conscious. Not only does it have specific functions, like running the autonomic nervous system, it also serves as a kind of clearinghouse and switching station where all sorts of sensory and motor pathways meet and connect and cross.

The cerebral cortex is the sheet of neurons that covers the two hemispheres of the brain. It is the "gray matter," the familiar, folded, lumpy-looking stuff everybody thinks of as "brain." Lifted off and spread out, the cerebral cortex would be about two and a half feet square and just a few millimeters thick—a slippery, not very attractive, but certainly unusual throw rug. What the cortex is wrapped around, besides the brainstem, is "white matter.'' White matter is made up of nerve cells of a type different from the ones that make up gray matter. The white matter cells function primarily as conductors of nerve impulses—like bundles of phone wires. Also beneath the cerebral cortex are the ventricles—four small, hollow cavities in the brain where cerebrospinal fluid is produced and stored. As its name implies, cerebrospinal fluid also fills the spinal canal.

All voluntary movement originates in the cerebral cortex and all sensory input registers there. Thinking and the production and comprehension of language are also functions of the cortex, and it plays a vital though less well understood role in memory and emotion as well.

There are two important principles that form the basis for the organization of the cerebral cortex. The first is the principle of contralateral control, by which the right side of the brain controls the left side of the body and the left side of the brain controls the right side of the body. The second is the principle of cerebral localization, according to which various functions of the brain are connected with specific sites on the cortex.

Although there are exceptions to all the rules, and no map of the cortex can be considered exact, enough is known about cerebral localization to make possible many connections between function and site. The visual cortex, for instance, is located at the back of the brain, while the language center is on the left side of the brain, in the temporal region. The frontal lobes, located just behind the forehead, are the newest part of the brain and the part that is unique to man. They are not nearly as well understood as some of the motor and sensory divisions of the cortex. Mood, personality, and emotion are some of the intangible products that have been connected with the frontal lobes.

As wonderful as the brain is, the spinal cord is almost as wonderful. A rope of nervous tissue no thicker than a fat pencil, the spinal cord is probably the single most overlooked, underrated piece of anatomy in the entire body. It's not as glamorous as the brain, it's a more utilitarian sort of a thing. People get so caught up thinking and worrying about their necks and their backs that they forget that their necks and their backs are one—the spinal column—and that inside the spinal column is the spinal cord, as delicate and organized and complicated as a direct extension of the brain ought to be. There is a tendency to cut things off at the head, to think of the brain as one thing and the rest of the body as another thing and let it go at that. But that is not the way it is. There is a little hole at the base of the skull, right at the top of the neck, called the foramen magnum. It is through the foramen magnum that the brain connects with the spinal cord. The spinal cord, just like the brain, is encased in bone. It is much smaller than the brain—the brain weighs about 1,500 grams, the spinal cord about 35 grams—but without it the brain is trapped.

Only about 45 centimeters long and one centimeter in diameter, the spinal cord is the pathway along which pass all the sensory information and the motor impulses that enable a human being to move his body and respond to his environment. In practice, while some of the surgical procedures performed on the brain are less delicate than others, every operation on the spinal cord is delicate because the cord is so densely packed with critical pathways. It is the spinal cord that joins the mind and the body and makes them one.

The nerves of the peripheral system are the fine branches radiating out into the body and the head from the spinal cord and the brain. (The peripheral nerves that originate in the brain are better known as the cranial nerves. There are twelve pairs of cranial nerves and they include the auditory nerves and the nerves that innervate the face.) There are two words to keep in mind when thinking about the spinal cord and the peripheral nervous system—*sensory* and *motor*. Sensory applies to all the information that comes into the peripheral system and travels back to the brain by way of the sensory pathways in the spinal cord. Motor impulses go the other way. They originate in the brain and then travel down the spinal cord, out into the peripheral system and on into the muscles by way of nerve cells known as motor neurons.

The autonomic nervous system connects with the brainstem both directly and by way of the spinal cord.

As noted, it handles involuntary functions like breathing and the beating of the heart, and it monitors and regulates the other vital organs, including the liver, the kidneys, and the sweat glands. It is also involved in sexual function. The autonomic nervous system consists of two parts—the sympathetic nervous system and the parasympathetic nervous system. The sympathetic system expends energy—it increases heart rate, stimulates the sweat glands, fires off the adrenal gland, and contracts the sphincter. When a dog leaps out of the bushes at you and you flee, that is your sympathetic system at work. The parasympathetic system is the opposite—it slows the heart rate and breathing. It is an energy-conserving system. The autonomic nervous system is connected with emotional response at a very basic level. A rage reaction is an autonomic function, as is its opposite, a state of serenity.

As good a way as any to get the nervous system established in your mind as a single entity is to snap your fingers. Just reach out . . . and snap your fingers. Do it again. Now do it with your other hand.

When you snap your fingers your nervous system is occupied as follows: Your brainstem is keeping you conscious, among many other functions. Your autonomic nervous system is keeping your heart beating and your lungs pumping. You are serene. You read a sentence that suggests that you snap your fingers. Your visual cortex receives the information from your optic nerve and sends it to the language center on your cortex, which interprets the message. You decide to snap your fingers.

When you snap your fingers with your right hand, the movement originates in what is called the motor strip on the left side of your brain. This motor strip—there is a matching one on the other side of your brain—is a narrow band of cortex that starts at about the top of your ear and runs up and over the top of the hemisphere and down into the fold between the two hemispheres, in the middle of your head. The motor strip has been mapped in great detail. Starting over your ear and moving up, it runs like this: larynx, tongue, lips, nostrils, eyelid, brow, neck, thumb, fingers, wrist, elbow, shoulder, trunk, hip, knee, leg, ankle, toes. So, when you snap the fingers on your right hand, the patch of cortex that's controlling the movement is about halfway between the top of your ear and the middle of your head. The impulse travels down through your brainstem, down the motor pathways of your spinal cord, out into your peripheral nervous system, down the nerves in your arm to the muscles in your fingers and—snap. Your auditory nerve then sends the sensory information on the sound to the auditory patch of your cortex, which analyzes it, and the gesture is complete. The central nervous system, the peripheral nervous system, and the autonomic nervous system, all in sync, are all working together as the human nervous system. Perfect, most of the time.

Part One

THE CUTTING EDGE

I

HISTORY

THE history of neurological medicine is gory and bizarre. It is also daring and noble. Like the human nervous system itself, it brings together the physical and the metaphysical, combining a search for empirical knowledge about the nervous system with an inquiry into the nature of the mind and the soul. A story that begins more than five thousand years ago and carries forward to the present age, it is marked by great breakthroughs and enduring mysteries, by the discovery of cures and of incurable diseases.

The story begins in disorder and moves toward order. In that classic trajectory it is like an individual case—something is wrong and knowledge is required to diagnose and treat the problem. But in contrast to an individual case, where usually only one thing is wrong, at the beginning of neurological history everything was wrong—the prehistoric human population was afflicted with a variety of neurological disorders and had no idea of what to do about any of them. It is fascinating and a little strange to speculate about the medical status of the earliest *Homo sapiens*. Logic holds that those peoples had an incidence of neurological and mental illness roughly equivalent to what has been found in the species over recorded time, and that raises the rather disturbing specter of schizophrenic cave men, epileptic cave men, cave men with brain tumors, cave men with Parkinson's disease. In addition to that, there was undoubtedly a lot of head, neck, and back trauma. With all that in mind, a simple statement is possible: the history of neurological medicine begins at the specific but unknown point in prehistoric time when some long-ago human being first set out to treat some fellow member of the race who was suffering from an organic or traumatic disorder of the nervous system.

Exactly what the first practitioner of neurological medicine did is a mystery—it was probably something simple, like packing clay into a fractured skull—and he probably made no connection between, let's say, his patient's left-side head wound and his right-side paralysis. But he got things started, and what we do know, and have a remarkable amount of evidence to prove, is that by the time of the Neolithic era, prehistoric men in Europe had developed a genuine knack and even a penchant for cutting holes in each other's skulls. They did it often, they did it well, and the survival rate was good.

We know that prehistoric trepanation was widespread in Europe, because Neolithic skulls with man-made holes in them have been found in Great Britain, France, Switzerland, Italy, Sweden, Denmark, Germany, Austria, Poland, Russia, Spain, and Portugal. We know that the subjects recovered, because the skulls show signs of healing and some have more than one hole. We know the procedure was common, because of the sheer number of altered skulls that have been discovered; out of 120 skulls found in a single dolmen in France, for example, 40 had man-made holes in them. And, because of what we know about the primitive tools in use at the time, it's possible to figure out how Neolithic trepanations were done.

It has been estimated that the procedure took at least half an hour. After slicing through the scalp, the Stone Age surgeon used a sharpened stone to scrape or bore a hole in the skull. The survival rates seem to indicate that those early neurosurgeons knew enough not to pierce the dura mater, the protective membrane that covers the brain. It's unlikely a person could avoid a deadly infection if he had the dura opened and his cortex laid bare while lying on the floor of a cave or in a clearing in the forest and then received a dressing made of grass or an animal skin. The holes in the skull were not small, either. Usually four or five centimeters in diameter, some were as large as thirteen centimeters across—just over five inches. Also, the holes were made in all parts of the skull.

Why Neolithic man cut holes in his skull isn't known. Although a few of the ancient skulls show evidence of skull fracture, most of them are normal but for the man-made defects. Which means that if there were medical reasons for the procedures, they did not usually involve traumatic injury. So what other medical problems would the Neolithic surgeons decide to treat with trepanation? It's possible they were cutting holes in the heads of people who complained of severe headache, people who had seizures, or people who reported aural or visual hallucinations. If they operated for severe headache caused by a brain tumor, then it's possible the resulting decompression relieved the headache. In such a case, what amounts to a cure would have been effected. The same cannot be said for operations undertaken to treat epilepsy or mental illness. What can be said about those cases, however, is that if primitive surgeons bored holes for epilepsy and mental illness, they had good instincts; they knew that their patients' problems originated inside their skulls, and cutting holes in those skulls constituted logical attempts to solve those problems.

Another possibility is that the Neolithic trepanations were performed for religious or magical reasons, if, for instance, the symptoms of mental illness, epilepsy, or certain brain tumors were interpreted as the work of evil spirits.

These Neolithic procedures are not nearly so far from today's neurosurgery as they might first appear. The chief difference is the amount of anatomical knowledge possessed by the operator. The Neolithic surgeon apparently knew enough not to pierce the dura and that was about it; he knew little about the brain itself other than that it was delicate and important. His procedure ended where the modern procedure really begins—with the opening of the skull. And yet, within the context of the time and

place they were performed, these ancient trepanations
were successful. The Neolithic surgeons lacked a knowledge of neuroanatomy, but they didn't need it. If they
were performing magical procedures, it was their knowledge of magic and spirits that was important. Whatever
they were up to, their patients survived. Had they attempted to remove a brainstem glioma they would have
failed, just as a modern neurosurgeon, without the background in magic of his prehistoric predecessor, would
surely fail to purge the evil spirits afflicting a Neolithic
schizophrenic. In that sense, prehistoric trepanations
"worked" the same way that modern neurosurgical procedures "work," by the direct application of existing
knowledge to the problems at hand.

The recorded history of the human nervous system begins with the Edwin Smith Papyrus, a collection of case
histories originally put together about 3500 B.C. (The papyrus is a 1700 B.C. copy of the original manuscript.)
The cases described in this ancient Egyptian document
chiefly concern injuries received in battle. Thirteen cases
of skull fracture are included, and the papyrus contains
the first recorded use of the word *brain*. Among the neurological symptoms described are aphasia, focal and general seizures, convulsions, hemiplegia, and bleeding from
the nose and the ears. Each case includes a description
of the wound, a diagnosis, a prognosis, and a course of
treatment. For example:

Instructions concerning a gaping wound in his head,
penetrating to the bone and perforating his skull.
If thou examinest a man having a gaping wound in
his head, penetrating to the bone and perforating his
skull; thou shouldst palpate his wound; shouldst thou
find him unable to look at his two shoulders and his
breast and suffering with stiffness in his back . . .
Thou shouldst say regarding him: "One having a
gaping wound in his head, penetrating to the bone and
perforating his skull, while he suffers with stiffness in
his neck. An ailment which I shall treat."
Now, after thou hast stitched it, thou shouldst lay

fresh meat upon his wound the first day. Thou shouldst not bind it. Moor him at his mooring stakes until the period of his injury passes by. Thou shouldst treat it afterward with grease, honey and lint every day, until he recovers.

A description of the brain itself is contained in a more serious case.

Instructions concerning a gaping wound in his head, penetrating to the bone, smashing the skull and rending open the brain of his skull.

If thou examinest a man having a gaping wound in his head, penetrating to the bone, smashing his skull, and rending open the brain of his skull, thou shouldst palpate his wound. Shouldst thou find that smash which is in his skull like those corrugations which form in molten copper, and something therein throbbing and fluttering under thy fingers, like the weak place of an infant's crown before it becomes whole—when it has happened there is no throbbing and fluttering under thy fingers until the brain of his skull is rent open and he discharges blood from both his nostrils and he suffers with stiffness in his neck . . .

Thou shouldst say: "An ailment not to be treated."

Beyond the treatment of trauma as outlined in the papyrus, and the treatment of headache pain, those ancient Egyptians made no substantial contributions to neurological medicine. They considered the heart to be the most vital organ, both as the seat of the soul and the origin of the mind's functions. Indeed, until the fifth century B.C., when Anaxagoras of Athens first asserted that the brain was the seat of the soul and intelligence, the big question was whether it was the heart or the liver that was the source of the "vital principle."

It is in the work of Hippocrates that clinical neurology begins. In his treatise on epilepsy, titled *On the Sacred Disease*, Hippocrates made clear his concept of the brain and its function. "The brain is the interpreter of consciousness," he wrote in 400 B.C. "Men ought to know that from the brain, and from the brain only, arise our pleasures, joys, laughter and jests, as well as our sorrows, pains, griefs, and tears. Through it, in particular, we think, see, hear, and distinguish the ugly from the beautiful, the bad from the good, the pleasant from the unpleasant. It is the same thing which makes us mad and delirious, inspires us with dread and fear, whether by night or by day, brings sleeplessness, inopportune mistakes, aimless anxieties, absent-mindedness, and acts that are contrary to habit. These things that we suffer all come from the brain, when it is not healthy. . . ."

On the Sacred Disease was a contribution to the field of clinical neurology not matched until the late nineteenth century. Hippocrates' achievement is even more amazing when you take into account the fact that he held to the then popular humoral theory of human physiology. According to that theory, there are four vital humors in the body—blood, phlegm, black bile, and yellow bile—and it is the various proportions and temperatures of these that determine the state of one's health. Elaborate systems by which the humors were generated and moved about in the body were described. The brain was considered a gland, and one of its functions was the secretion of phlegm as a cooling agent. Its most important role, though, was as the site where the "pneuma," the essential element of life derived from the air, was introduced into the blood so that it could be distributed throughout the body. It was the presence of pneuma in the blood that made all movement and sensation possible. "When a man draws breath into himself," Hippocrates wrote, "the air first reaches the brain and so is dispersed through the rest of his body, though it leaves in the brain its quintessence, and all that it has of intelligence or sense."

That Hippocrates was able to come up with as much valid neurology as he did while holding such theories is testament to his skills as a clinician. His pure powers of observation are even more striking when you note that, because the Greeks were averse to the dissection of the human body, the only brains Hippocrates dissected were those of goats. Even though he believed that epilepsy was caused by phlegm that got into veins leading to the head and blocked the flow of air to the brain, his detailed descriptions of epileptic seizures of various types still constitute a valuable though precocious contribution to medical literature. He was even aware of the "aura" and the feeling of premonition that precede some epileptic seizures, and he described how some people would "know beforehand when they were about to be seized and flee from men either to their homes or to a deserted place and cover themselves up."

Besides discussion of epilepsy, Hippocrates' writings are filled with descriptions of a variety of other neurological disorders and symptoms, including hemiplegia, aphasia, migraine headaches, and sciatica. He recognized the concept of contralateral control, warning that incisions in the brain could cause convulsions on the opposite side of the body. He also displayed an understanding of strokes, pointing to numbness as one sign of an impending stroke and noting that "persons are most subject to apoplexy between the ages of forty and sixty."

Hippocrates' recognition of the brain as the seat of consciousness, movement, and sensation was the most important aspect of a tremendous overall achievement in medicine. "Neither, in truth, do I count it a worthy opinion to hold that the body of man is polluted by God," he wrote in *On the Sacred Disease* as he refuted the superstitions that had grown up around epilepsy. "This disease seems to me to be nowise more divine than others; but it has its nature such as other diseases have, and a cause when it originates." What Hippocrates did was declare disease a natural process, arising in the patient's body. He gave the physician his place in the world—at the patient's side, watching and thinking.

Hippocrates' work in neurology was not automatically accepted. Aristotle, the leading figure of the next generation, went on to a historic life as philosopher, biologist, and all-around genius while believing that the heart was the organ of intellect and the brain was merely a cooling device.

In Alexandria, Egypt, during the third century B.C., dissection of the human body began to be performed regularly, and one result was the first real progress in neuroanatomy. Herophilus of Chalcedon, considered the founder of the study of human anatomy, dissected hundreds of bodies. He recognized the brain as the organ of intellect and described it in some detail. He was the first to divide nerves into sensory and motor classifications and to describe the ventricles.

Eristratus of Chios was in Alexandria at about the same time, and his work has earned him recognition as the father of physiology. Comparing human brains with animal brains, he noted the convolutions of man's brain were more numerous and connected this with man's superior intelligence. Eristratus provided an elaborate theory of brain function. Air, or pneuma, went from the lungs to the heart, where it was changed into vital spirits. In the brain, the vital spirits were changed into animal spirits in the ventricles, and the animal spirits were then carried to the rest of the body through the nerves, which he believed were hollow. These animal spirits made movement possible.

Most of what we know about Eristratus and Herophilus comes from the writings of Galen of Pergamus, a Roman physician who studied in Alexandria in the second century A.D. and who built on and greatly expanded the work of his predecessors. Over the course of his long and extraordinary career, Galen wrote more than four hundred treatises and established himself as one of the most important figures in the history of medicine. Founder of experimental physiology, physician to gladiators, famous citizen of Rome, he was an egocentric philosopher whose belief in teleology and in his own infallibility helped stunt the growth of medicine, which his own scientific observations should have spurred. Galen was a medical genius up to his elbows in gore. Human dissection was once again taboo by his time, even in Alexandria, but his work with the gladiators provided him with plenty of head and spinal cord trauma and exposures. In addition, he was an enthusiastic vivisectionist whose work with animals included exploring the brains of live, unanesthetized goats, pigs, and apes. Writing about it, he said that he preferred to do such work on goats and pigs because that way ''you

avoid seeing the unpleasing expression of the ape when
it is vivisected."

Clinically, Galen's broad concepts of nervous system
disorders are more notable than his understanding of specific afflictions. From clinical observation he made the
simple but critical distinction between disorders of the
brain itself, like apoplexy, and disorders of brain function, like epilepsy. He also deduced that some local disorders, like partial paralysis, originate not in the brain
but in the spinal cord. Such conclusions are extraordinary, given the fact that Galen had no understanding of
cerebral localization.

Galen's overall theory of nervous system function was
an elaboration of the "spirits" concept, according to
which blood was produced in the liver, where digested
food and the "natural spirits" were combined. The blood
then went to the right side of the heart for purification
and from there to the left side of the heart, where it was
invested with "vital spirits." From the heart, some of
the blood went to the rest of the body and some of it
went to the brain. The blood that went to the brain circulated in the area around the pituitary gland, where the
"vital spirits" were transformed into "animal spirits,"
a process that also involved the cerebral ventricles. These
"animal spirits" were then carried throughout the body
by the nerves and were the source of all nervous system
activity.

There are two important points about Galen's concept
of nervous system function. One attests to the breadth of
his vision, the other defines its limits. On the one hand,
his basic idea of a form of energy flowing from the brain
through the rest of the body is pretty close to the truth. On
the other, the structure that he considered most critical
in the transformation of "vital spirits" into "animal spirits," a web of tiny blood vessels called the rete mirabile,
is found in the brains of oxen but not in humans.

After Galen, little progress was made until the Renaissance. The most notable neurological concept developed during the pre-Renaissance period was the
localization of all mental faculties in the ventricles of
the brain. Nemesius, one of the Fathers of the Church of

the fourth century A.D., proposed that sensation and imagination originated in the anterior ventricle, for sensual perception was the first step in thinking; reason and intellect, where information was analyzed, originated in the middle ventricle; and memory, where selected images and ideas were retained, was the province of the posterior ventricle. Not even Galen, who had defined the elements of the soul in roughly the same way, had gone so far as to give them specific locations in the brain. And the Fathers of the Church did it without the benefit of any fresh research. Since the ventricles were *places* in the brain but not actually *parts* of the brain, the theory neatly avoided certain sticky metaphysical problems. It enabled believers in the noncorporeal soul to account for human behavior without assigning the immaterial functions of the mind and soul to mere human tissue.

Crude illustrations of the human head with the various sections appropriately marked were circulated widely for hundreds of years, and the simple theory became the definitive account of the workings of the mind. Not until the sixteenth century, when Andreas Vesalius of Brussels pointed out the presence of ventricles in a variety of dumb animals, thereby eliminating any exclusive connection between the ventricles and the highest functions of the human mind, did this theory crumble.

It was Vesalius who elevated the study of human anatomy to a science. Educated at Louvain, Montpellier, and Paris, he became a professor of surgery and anatomy at the University of Padua in 1537, at the age of twenty-three. Vesalius was a true Renaissance figure who made the most of the artistic and intellectual freedom of the times. Free to perform all the dissections he wanted to in the stimulating environment of Padua, which drew students from all over Europe, Vesalius dedicated himself to the task of accurately and objectively describing the anatomy of the human body. Though he was a Galenist and adhered to most of the Greek's theories of nervous system function, Vesalius was not interested in fitting his findings to established theories or proposing new theories; rather, he wanted to look, see, and describe what he saw as clearly as possible.

In 1543, at the age of twenty-nine, Vesalius published a seven-volume work called *De humani corporis fabrica*, known as the Fabrica. With extraordinary engravings by Jan Kalkar, who had studied with Titian, the Fabrica opened up the human body and showed it to the world. One of the finest products of the Renaissance, and possibly the best medical text ever published, the Fabrica divides the history of medicine in two: the time before it was published, when the study of human anatomy was disorganized and speculative; and the time after it was published, when the study of human anatomy followed a scientific approach and became more solidly based on fact.

One of the seven volumes of the Fabrica dealt with the overall anatomy of the nervous system, and another dealt exclusively with the brain. Vesalius described the brain and the nervous system more accurately and in more detail than they had ever been described before. The fifteen illustrations by Kalkar that were included in the volume on the brain remain stunning to this day, not merely for their incredible anatomic detail but for their beauty. They do for the brain what Vesalius did for the human body—they do it justice.

Vesalius was not the only seminal neuroanatomist to adhere to strange concepts of neurophysiology while making great breakthroughs in the study of the anatomy of the brain and the nervous system. Thomas Willis, who in 1664 published *Cerebri anatomi*, the next classic text in neuroanatomy after the Fabrica, was also a believer in "animal spirits" as the prime source of nervous system activity. Willis, the most successful London physician of his time, was the first to use the term *neurology*. He was an industrious researcher and clinician who made a major contribution to knowledge of the nervous system. But his genius for observation was marred by a flair for concocting erroneous theories of nervous system function. While deducing the existence of the autonomic nervous system, he mistakenly located it in the cerebellum: "When some time past I diligently and seriously meditated on the Office of the Cerebel . . . this true and genuine use of it occurred; to wit, that the cerebel is a peculiar fountain of animal spirits designed for some works, and wholly distinct from the Brain . . . the Office of the Cerebel seems to be for the animal Spirits to supply some Nerves, by which involuntary actions (such as are the beating of the heart, easie respiration, the Concoctions of the aliment, the protrusion of the Chyle, and many others) which are made after a constant manner unknown to us, or whether we will or no, are performed.'' Similarly, when he decided that memory was lodged in the cerebral cortex, he supported his theory by pointing out: ''For as often as we endeavour to remember objects long since past, we rub the Temples and forepart of the Head.''

However, it would be a mistake to think of Willis merely as a man burdened with a bad understanding of physiology. The twist is that he made many excellent observations even while believing in ''animal spirits.'' It was he who revised Galen's description of the cranial nerves, and he was the first to use the terms *hemisphere* and *lobe* in describing the brain. In his own way, he also addressed the subject of psychiatric disorders, writing at length on cases of hysteria, melancholia, and manic depression. In a passage distinguishing ''stupidity'' and ''foolishness,'' Willis is said by some to have produced the first description of schizophrenia; ''For those affected with [foolishness] apprehend simple things well enough, dextrously and swiftly, and retain them firm in their memory, but by reason of a defect of judgement, they compose or divide their notions evilly, and very badly infer one thing from another.''

While knowledge of the anatomy of the brain and nervous system accumulated, knowledge of their physiology lagged behind. What was missing was an understanding of the basic mechanism of nervous system function, the nerve impulse, and of the underlying role of electricity in the nervous system. It was the work of Luigi Galvani of Bologna in the 1700s that finally put an end to the ''animal spirits'' theory of nervous system function. One day Galvani noticed that some frog legs hanging on copper hooks from an iron balcony were twitching. Examining this phenomenon in a series of experiments, Galvani established the concept of "animal electricity." Publishing his findings in 1791, he declared that it was electricity and not "animal spirits" that flowed through the nervous system.

By the beginning of the nineteenth century, after hundreds of years of groping research and bolts of inspiration, a lot of details about the anatomy and functions of the human nervous system had been discovered. But the pieces of the puzzle hadn't been put together; in fact, some very important pieces were still missing and wouldn't be found for decades. Nevertheless there was, as there had always been, a strong desire on the part of some neurological researchers to build their slim knowledge into a larger theory of brain function. This drive was never more completely or more strangely submitted to than by Franz Joseph Gall. Gall, born in 1758, was a leading neuroanatomist who, among other things, was the first to establish the distinction between the white matter and the gray matter of the brain. Working in Vienna with his associate Johann Christoph Spurzheim, Gall produced a four-volume work on the anatomy of the nervous system that included one hundred copper-plate illustrations. It was his masterpiece, and it was based on the solid scientific concept of direct observation. But Gall was not content with the objective rigors of anatomical research. He could not help but notice the tantalizing distance between the slippery gore he picked over in the laboratory and the endless complexity and variety of human behavior. Gall wanted to close that distance, so he made one of the great theoretical leaps in the history of medicine.

Franz Gall was the first to formulate in detail an essentially correct theory of cerebral localization. Cerebral localization is probably the most important concept in the development of modern neurology. Gall began with the phenomenon of individuality. He wondered why some people behaved one way and some another. Some people were intelligent, others stupid. Some were kind, others murderers. He concluded that all human behavior was the result of "faculties" that were developed to varying degrees in each individual. He listed twenty-seven—later

thirty-seven—such faculties and declared that they were
functions of the brain. Specifically, he said, for each fac-
ulty there was a corresponding "organ," and those organs together made up the cerebral cortex. Each organ
had an exact location in the brain, and that location was
the same for every human being. However, the degree to
which the various faculties and their related organs were
developed was different in each case. Hence, individuality. Gall backed his claims with proof based on com-
parative anatomy.

For Gall, then, the brain was not merely a gland or a
sensory receptor; it was the organic source of the mental
and emotional life of man, and its anatomic development
was the thing that separated man from all other animals.
One respectful historian has written that Gall "gave a
new dignity to the brain" when he made it the source of
the "faculties." That's true, but Gall got carried away
with his theory and said that each organ was in turn manifest in the contours of the skull and that the degree of
development of the organs could be determined by a
careful examination of the skull. In other words, the
bumps on a person's head were a direct reflection of his
personality, and if one knew the system one could do a
full personality analysis. Gall said that he first got the
idea of faculties and their physical manifestations when
he was a schoolboy and noticed that the students with
the best memories all seemed to have bulging eyes.

Gall called his system "anatomical personology," but
it became popular as "phrenology." What's most intriguing about Gall's concept of localization is the rather
cavalier way he passed over the more mundane motor and
sensory functions and instead located elusive intellectual
and moral phenomena like sexual love, ambition, wit,
courage, and even "attraction to wine." He produced
elaborate charts and traveled throughout Europe demonstrating and promoting his controversial ideas. He went
so far as to examine the heads of statues of famous persons like Caesar and Napoleon. His associate, Spurzheim, brought phrenology to the United States. Because
it reduced the complexity of the human mind to the sim-
plicity of a road map, phrenology had great appeal and

it made Gall a rich man, but it cost him his reputation as a scientist, and the controversy over his ideas forced him out of Vienna. He died in Paris in 1828. Ironically, his skull was preserved and remains today part of the collection of the Musée de l'Homme in Paris. It is unremarkable in appearance.

In its sheer reach, Gall's theory echoed man's perennial search for the seat of the soul. For Aristotle, the soul was in the heart. Plato located the immortal soul in the head and the two parts of the mortal soul in the chest and the belly. In the seventeenth century the French philosopher René Descartes concluded that the soul was located in the pineal gland, a tiny, unpaired structure near the center of the brain. At one time or another, others have located the soul in the ventricles of the brain and even in the cerebrospinal fluid. So powerful is the idea of the seat of the soul that even modern anatomists cannot wholly ignore it. In *The Human Brain*, his 1981 anatomy book, John Nolte noted, "Since each of us has only one pineal gland, which is located deep within the brain, it was thought for a time that this organ might be the seat of the soul. This now *seems unlikely* [emphasis added], since pineal tumors do not cause the changes one would expect to find associated with distortion of the soul." A variation on the search for the seat of the soul that was actively pursued for many years was a search for the sensorium commune—a single site where all sensory information is received and processed.

In retrospect, Gall's work places him in a murky zone between the earlier yearnings to locate the soul and the later, successful attempts to locate certain motor and sensory functions in the brain. He was the last of a long line of speculators and theorists who, because of limited anatomical and physiological knowledge, relied on their imaginations to account for the fabulous workings of the human nervous system.

In the thirty-three years following Gall's death, knowledge of the human nervous system exploded as microscopy and laboratory techniques for fixing and staining tissues advanced rapidly. In the late 1830s, the neuron was seen for the first time, and by the 1860s, it had been described roughly as we know it today. The concept of reflex action, critical to understanding the relationships of the various parts of the nervous system and for making clinical diagnoses, was established, and the anatomy and physiology of the spinal cord were receiving their first serious attention. The essential details of the autonomic nervous system were also discovered during this time. Ironically, one of the few things in neurology that didn't progress during those years was the theory of cerebral localization, which had been "disproved" by the French anatomist Marie-Jean-Pierre Flourens in the 1820s. Then, in 1861, another Frenchman, Pierre-Paul Broca, reported on a case of aphasia, and the golden age of neurology got under way.

Broca's establishment of a motor speech center on the left side of the brain signaled a renewed interest in cerebral localization. In 1870, a series of breakthrough experiments by two German researchers was reported. Edward Hitzig and Gustav Theodor Fritsch used platinum electrodes to explore the cerebral cortexes of dogs. Using a weak charge, the two established the existence of motor centers in the brain. Their work was built upon almost immediately by the Englishman Sir David Ferrier, who refined the system for cortical stimulation and achieved remarkably discrete motor function demonstrations in a variety of animals, including rabbits, pigeons, and monkeys. In 1874, the German neurologist Carl Wernicke published a classic monograph describing sensory aphasia, which has since come to be known as Wernicke's aphasia. Wernicke went on to identify almost all of the major pieces of the language puzzle as we know it today. Two years after Wernicke's monograph, Ferrier published his book *The Functions of the Brain*, and the theory of cerebral localization effectively became the principle of cerebral localization. The basic wiring of the human nervous system was understood.

From the time of Hippocrates until the second half of the nineteenth century, neurological disorders were not diagnosed, they were merely described. Some of the de-

scriptions were better than others—in 1817, James Parkinson described "shaking palsy" so well that the disease was eventually named after him—but for the most
part it was a matter of fitting disorders into a few broad
categories. The general groupings were the same for cen-
turies: apoplexy, epilepsy, mental illness, movement disorders, and sensory disorders. Once a physician had
described and classified a neurological disease, he usually prescribed whatever medicines and methods were in
general use at the time. At the end of the eighteenth century, for instance, epilepsy was treated with valerian (an
herb root) and phosphorus; melancholia was treated with
camphor and opium; insanity, with belladonna. Heroic
purgation and bleeding were undertaken in cases where
it was believed that the nervous disease was due to irri-
tation of the gastrointestinal tract. Of course, there were
also always quacks about, and some of their neurological
treatments were inspired. In the sixteenth century, quacks
declared that insanity and other mental disturbances were
caused by stones in the head. Their solution was simple—
neurosurgery. After cutting the scalp, the quack surgeon
simply palmed a few rocks, "removed" them from the
patient's head, showed them to any interested family
members, and then dropped them noisily into a bucket.

Clinical neurology finally surged forward in the years
between 1860 and 1900, driven primarily by the work of
two men—John Hughlings Jackson in England and Jean-
Martin Charcot in France—as well as major new developments in anatomy, physiology, and pathology. Charcot
and Jackson created modern clinical neurology by applying the new ideas to the diagnosis and, to a lesser extent,
to the treatment of neurological disorders.

After 1862, when, at thirty-six, he was appointed its
chief physician, Charcot lived out his professional life
literally surrounded by patients in the wards of the enormous general hospital Salpêtrière, which had been built
in 1603 as an arsenal before being made into a home for
abandoned old women and, later, an insane asylum. It
was a huge complex of some forty-five buildings, and in
its population of five thousand ravaged patients, Charcot
could find examples of just about every nervous system

disease. He was a hands-on physician who made his reputation at the side of his patients. His genius was for clinical observation and for teaching.

Charcot didn't so much see his patients as illuminate them. Their nervous systems, and the diseases that altered their natural flow, lit up under his remarkable gaze. He created a system of labs—pathology, microscopy, photography, anatomical drawing and sculpture—to back up his work in the wards. Because of his attention to clinical detail, the list of neurological disorders became longer and more exact. Among his many accomplishments, he was the first to identify ALS, amyotrophic lateral sclerosis (Lou Gehrig's disease). He was also the first to establish, through clinical examination, the existence of a motor strip on the cortex of man; before Charcot the motor strip had been demonstrated only on animals in research labs. Charcot also played an important role in the development and refinement of the neurological exam. And he raised the education of medical students to the level of art—theatrical art, to be exact. Charcot's weekly sessions in a six-hundred-seat auditorium at Salpêtrière were virtuoso performances in which the master physician would sit on the stage and demonstrate various diseases and symptoms in patients, the setting dramatically lit for maximum effect. What Charcot did, in sum, was to create the very first department of neurology, complete with all the major components, and in running it he set the standard for the practice of clinical neurology.

Jackson, like Charcot, was an incisive clinician, and his work with epilepsy and aphasia at the National Hospital for the Paralysed and Epileptic in London was groundbreaking. Strictly through clinical observation, he anticipated in detail the concept of cerebral localization as it was eventually established in the labs. Ferrier's book on the subject, in fact, includes clinical material supplied by Jackson. Jackson's elaborate analysis of the nature and variety of seizures is the foundation upon which all subsequent studies of epilepsy are based. But, as important as Jackson's clinical work was, he has a place in history for his ability to think about the nervous system as much as for his ability to diagnose its disorders.

* * *

The modern age of neurosurgery began on November 25, 1884, at the National Hospital for the Paralysed and Epileptic in Regent's Park, London, when Sir Rickman John Godlee and A. Hughes Bennett removed a tumor from the brain of a twenty-five-year-old Scottish farmer. It was a landmark case because it was the first time a brain tumor had been removed after being diagnosed and located with the newly developed principle of cerebral localization. The patient's symptoms included increasing weakness of the left arm and left-sided convulsions. Godlee opened the skull over the right motor strip and, after opening the dura, found the tumor just below the surface of the brain. He removed it with a surgical spoon.

The importance of the Regent's Park operation is certified by the remarkable group of observers on hand for it: Jackson, Ferrier, and Sir Victor Horsley (who would shortly establish himself as one of the best of the first generation of brain surgeons). The operation's legendary status is such that some of the conversation that took place has been reported. At the end of the operation, Hughlings Jackson turned to David Ferrier and said, "Awful, awful." Ferrier protested that the operation had gone very well. "Yes," Jackson replied, "but he opened a Scotsman's head and failed to put a joke in it." The Scotsman did well for a while but then developed meningitis and died within a month, an unfortunate fact that did nothing to erode the operation's importance.

The operation successfully brought together the booming field of neurology and the recently civilized field of surgery. Prior to the development of anesthesia in the 1840s, surgery was a brutal process in which the prime requirements was speed. A patient might be rendered stuporous with whiskey, knocked out by pressure on the carotid artery, or merely "mesmerized" before being restrained on the operating table. Then the surgeon would do his work as quickly as possible—amputations that took less than a minute were the standard. With the introduction of ether and chloroform as anesthetic agents, surgery took a great leap forward, but it remained a bad business because of the high infection rate. A surgery patient in the mid-nineteenth century who survived the operation stood a good chance of dying of gangrene or some other bacterial infection. In 1866, with Joseph Lister's development of the antiseptic technique, surgery was finally lifted out of the darkness. With anesthesia and the antiseptic technique (which rapidly gave way to the more effective aseptic technique) surgeons could attempt more complicated and more time-consuming procedures. For the first time, something beyond simple trepanation was possible; cranial surgery could become intracranial surgery, and brain surgery could begin to emerge as a valid specialty.

Lister himself concluded that surgery of the brain was possible after attempting to remove a brain tumor prior to the Godlee-Bennett operation. Operating on a patient who exhibited the symptoms of a tumor on the right side of the brain, he trephined over the right frontal lobe. When he lifted away the bone the brain bulged out of the opening in the skull. Lister explored the protruding brain with his finger, rupturing a ventricle in the process. He failed to find the tumor, but the rupture caused the brain to decompress, and the patient improved briefly before lapsing into a coma and dying eight days later. At autopsy, Lister discovered that his finger had missed the tumor by only half an inch. It was the way that the wound in the head healed postoperatively that convinced Lister that brain surgery was possible.

One of the biggest problems these surgeons faced was the medical community's widespread opinion that brain tumors were untreatable. If they were treated at all, brain tumors were usually treated as symptoms of syphilis; mercury and potassium iodide were rubbed on the patient's head, often for months, with patients sometimes going blind from the treatment. It was the surgeons' position that the key to successful brain tumor operations was early diagnosis, but the prevailing belief that brain tumors meant sure death was not easily overcome, and resistance to the new specialty persisted. As a result, there was little change in the grim prognosis for all patients with brain tumors, and the mortality rates among the first groups of surgery patients were extremely high.

Mortality rates from 55 percent to over 90 percent were reported in the first twenty-five years of the specialty, and many of the deaths were no doubt due to the fact that the operations were performed too late. By the time they were diagnosed and the decision was made to try surgery, the tumors were so large nothing could save the patients. As crude as the early techniques were, it was the slowness with which the medical community changed its attitudes about brain tumors that kept brain surgery as a treatment of last resort for so very long.

Which is not to say that the specialty arrived full blown. Even with anesthesia and the antiseptic and aseptic techniques, surgery in the late 1800s was a risky, dirty business by current standards. Lighting was poor. The application of the anesthetic agents was inexact, and there was no systematic monitoring of heartbeat, respiration, or blood pressure. The extent of the sterile field was minimal, and the surgeons operated without caps, masks, or even gloves. Occasionally they operated without gowns, in their street clothes.

The accepted methods for handling the exposed brain and removing brain tumors were also rather crude. William W. Keen, who performed the first brain tumor operation in the United States, in 1887, was consistent with the approach of the times when he recommended in 1892 that brain tumors be scooped out with the finger. If it wasn't possible to use the finger, Keen suggested a knife, scissors, a sharp spoon, or an ordinary teaspoon. Keen also used the handle of a plain teaspoon for retracting the brain during an operation. Generally, it was the practice to remove brain tumors as quickly as possible. Because the localization of tumors was not exact, tumors that were below the surface of the cortex were sometimes pinpointed by the repeated insertion of a long needle into the brain. Various devices were created to enable the surgeons to locate the points on the scalp that corresponded to the major anatomical features of the brain. One of these, devised in 1888, consisted of a curved metal bar that went over the patient's head and a sliding bar with marked settings for the different parts of the brain. In the case of tumors that could not be localized or were too

deep in the brain to be operable, a palliative procedure
was often performed for the purpose of decompression.
In these cases, the surgeon would simply open the scalp,
remove a piece of the skull, and then close the scalp. The
operation became quite popular, for it decreased intracranial pressure and provided the patients with real
relief. The main drawback was the way the brain bulged
out of the opening in the skull and made a large, ugly
lump on the patient's head.

These procedures sound primitive because they were
primitive, but it would be a mistake and an injustice to
dismiss the early years of neurosurgery as some kind of
long-running medical freak show. Those first brain surgeons were doing things that had never been done before
and they were losing a lot of patients in the process. But
in the long run they made a tremendous contribution.
They and their patients were paying a large and bloody
initiation fee into a new age in medicine and surgery.

The man who made neurosurgery into a modern medical specialty was Harvey Williams Cushing. Again, the
story is order out of disorder, and no man created more
order in those antique operating rooms than Cushing. He
transformed the practice of brain surgery from a quasi-
experimental oddity into a valid therapeutic science and
an art. In the process, he created a new surgical standard
for all fields and defined the role of the brain surgeon as
a fastidious technician. He was the father of modern neurosurgery.

Cushing was born in Cleveland in 1869. His father,
grandfather, and great-grandfather were all physicians,
as was his older brother Edward. He did his undergraduate work at Yale and graduated from Harvard Medical
School in 1895. As a medical student and then as a resident at the Massachusetts General Hospital, Cushing became well acquainted with the state of surgery in the
1890s and he was not impressed. In his second year of
medical school, he began administering anesthesia during operations. The techniques were crude—sea sponges
soaked in ether were applied directly—and there was no
monitoring during the course of the operation. In 1893,

Cushing lost a patient while handling the anesthesia in front of a class of fellow students. Such deaths were not uncommon, but shortly after his experience Cushing and another student, Amory Codman, devised a chart for keeping track of the pulse and respiratory rates of patients during surgery. It was a simple yet critically important innovation and it set the pattern for Cushing's career, reflecting a dissatisfaction with the status quo and a respect for detail. It may well be that the contribution Cushing made as a precocious medical student was his greatest. The use of ether charts, as they were known, evolved, spread rapidly, and ultimately improved every surgical procedure performed from then on.

Cushing witnessed only a few neurosurgical procedures as a medical student, and none of them were particularly successful; two craniotomies he assisted on in the summer of 1895 were both fatalities. But his interest in the field grew, and in 1901, while taking a year off from his duties as a surgeon at Johns Hopkins University, Cushing toured Europe and visited several of the top European neurologists and surgeons. His visit to Victor Horsley was brief but notable. Cushing accompanied Horsley on a daring house call. After washing up at his own home and wrapping his instruments in a towel for the carriage ride to the patient's house, the Englishman proceeded to perform a craniotomy and a cranial nerve dissection for relief of facial nerve pain. According to one account of the event, Horsley had his patient under ether in five minutes, the operation under way in fifteen minutes, and the whole thing over with in less than an hour. Cushing was horrified and gave up on a plan to study with the master of British neurosurgery. He had more rewarding experiences with doctors in France and Switzerland, but on the whole he found the conditions in the hospitals and operating rooms of Europe to be poor.

Near the end of his trip, Cushing was in Liverpool and took part in some extraordinary experiments being conducted by Sir Charles Scott Sherrington, known as the founder of modern neurophysiology. "It does not come within the realm of everyday experience to be called upon to trephine a gorilla," Cushing wrote in his diary. Sherrington was researching cerebral localization. In three days the two men opened the skulls and stimulated the motor strips of an orangutan, a chimpanzee, and a gorilla. These were long, strange sessions—eight- and nine-hour days of probing the anthropoid brains with electrodes, watching the twitching limbs of the heavily etherized primates, and mapping their exposed cortexes. During the gorilla experiment, one assistant kept a revolver handy, Cushing noted, ''so that if it came to the worst, there would be no scandal.''

Back in the United States, Cushing positioned himself as a specialist in neurological surgery. Between 1902 and 1907 he performed thirty-nine brain tumor operations at Johns Hopkins, with little success. But, despite the fact that few in the medical community, including his old friend Codman, considered the surgical removal of brain tumors feasible, Cushing persevered. He developed an operation for the treatment of trigeminal neuralgia, a disorder of the fifth cranial nerve that causes severe, even disabling facial pain. At the same time, he was operating on the spinal cord. In 1904, Cushing presented his first paper on neurological surgery, and four years later he was asked to contribute an eighty-page chapter on surgery of the head for a five-volume work on surgery. Cushing turned in a heavily illustrated eight-hundred-page manuscript. Eventually published as a book of less than half the length, Cushing's text established neurosurgery as a specialty.

Cushing remained the central figure in the development of neurosurgery until his death in 1939. His contributions range from the invention of electrocautery to the practice of shaving patients at the last moment before operating to avoid infection. In 1901, Cushing introduced in the United States a pneumatic device for the measurement of blood pressure that he had come upon while touring Italy. In just a few years, the monitoring of blood pressure during surgery was standard procedure. He also developed many mechanical aids, including a special tourniquet for controlling bleeding of the scalp and various clips for blood vessels. He produced five volumes on brain tumors, including a 1932 classification of tumors that was drawn from the more than two thousand confirmed cases he had operated on. His case histories are famous for their thoroughness, usually including photographs and sketches of the operations by Cushing himself. Cushing maintained a lifelong interest in the pituitary gland. When he accomplished the rare feat of identifying a new disease—now called Cushing's disease—it was a disorder of the pituitary gland. His research into the subject included trips to circus side shows, where he would examine and take the histories of the giants, dwarfs, fat ladies, and other "freaks" on display. One summer, when his family went away on vacation, he moved a group of dwarfs into his home in order to test a growth hormone on them. But Cushing's largest contribution to the development of neurosurgery was simply his approach. He was a slow, careful surgeon, a tyrant in the operating room who would allow no sloppiness, and he brought all surgery into the twentieth century, by will power as much as anything else.

Of course, Cushing was not the only brain surgeon at work in those years. The specialty progressed through the efforts of many surgeons. Highlights in that progress include the development of ventriculography in 1918 by Walter Edward Dandy, a technical master who had studied under Cushing. A diagnostic technique important in the location of brain tumors, ventriculography was a dangerous business that involved drilling small holes in the skull and then injecting air into the ventricles of the brain. X rays then revealed any distortion of the ventricles caused by a tumor. Nine years later, another critical diagnostic procedure was introduced by the Portuguese brain surgeon António Egas Moniz. Cerebral angiography, which is still in wide use today, enabled surgeons to see the blood supply of the brain on X ray. Moniz's technique, which has been refined considerably, involved the injection of a solution of sodium iodide directly into the carotid artery, which he exposed during an operation.

As might be expected, World War I was a key factor in the development of neurosurgery, as it was in the development of all medicine. In just a few years, the surgeons involved were exposed to a lifetime's worth of nervous system trauma. Unfortunately, individual case records were not always well kept under the battlefield conditions, and bureaucratic resistance foiled Cushing's dream of a national file that would have brought together all the information that was accumulated.

During the 1930s, the education and training of neurosurgeons became more formalized. In earlier years, most neurosurgeons were simply general surgeons who developed an interest in the nervous system and pursued it; but by the end of the 1930s, the first residency programs had been put in place. The 1930s also saw the publication of Hans Berger's landmark works on the electrical activity of the brain. Berger identified the alpha and beta waves, the two major electrical rhythms of the brain, and created the science of the electroencephalograph (EEG).

In the 1940s, although brain surgery was benefiting from the ever-improving residency programs as well as the harsh experience of World War II, it was still a primitive business. The level of crudeness is documented in *Death Be Not Proud*, John Gunther's book about the death of his son John, Jr., from a brain tumor at the age of seventeen. Because decompression was still standard procedure, when the surgeons operated on Gunther's son, they left out a chunk of his skull so that the brain would not be squeezed as the tumor grew back. As a result, the boy spent the final months of his life with a tennis-ball-size bulge protruding from his head. Gunther wrote, "The flap, which we called the Bulge or the Bump, got slowly, mercilessly bigger."

In the 1950s, operative techniques continued to improve. The development of corticosteroids enabled doctors to control swelling of the brain during and after surgery. Along with more careful and complete tumor removal, artificial steroids brought an end to the use of decompression as a treatment. The invention of the ventricular shunt for the treatment of hydrocephalus (water on the brain) was another critical achievement of that time. Tens of thousands of shunts have been placed in people's brains over the last thirty years, and the operation is almost routinely successful.

In the 1960s, the introduction of the operative microscope by the Swiss neurosurgeon Gazi Yasargil completely transformed vascular surgery of the nervous
system—the operative treatment of aneurysms and arteriovenous malformations (AVMS)—and made all neurosurgical procedures, including tumor operations, more
exact. The microscope took neurosurgeons deeper into
the nervous system than ever before and created new
standards of success across the board.

The current era of neurosurgery began with the invention of the CAT (computerized axial tomography) scanner in the early 1970s, and the subsequent development
of the PET (positronemission tomography) scanner and
magnetic resonance imaging (MRI). Today, a thirty-six-
year-old neurosurgeon qualifies roughly as a member of
his specialty's fifth generation and can claim Harvey
Cushing as his professional great-great-grandfather. The
second century of brain surgery is under way.

II

HOSPITAL

From the balcony outside the fourteenth floor of the Neurological Institute of New York the world is a large and busy place. To the south stretches the buzzing clutter of the island of Manhattan, jetliners banking low over its miles of rooftops, its familiar midtown skyline hazy in the distance, more than 120 blocks away. Immediately to the west runs the wide and powerful Hudson River, close enough for the names of the tankers and freighters that constantly ply it to be easily made out. To the north, just ten blocks away, the George Washington Bridge hums with endless traffic. To the east, barely seen, lie the reaches of the Bronx, Queens, and Long Island, laced with highways, parkways, and expressways, home to two major airports. Straight down are the noisy and crowded streets of the neighborhood known as Washington Heights, where the sound of sirens is common and where, at the corner of 168th Street and Broadway, sidewalk entrepreneurs sell toys and flowers to people on their way to visit patients at the huge Columbia Presbyterian Medical Center.

Altogether, the view from the balcony is like a picture from an old civics studies text, the one illustrating the chapter on cities. It evokes a sense of the population of New York going about its collective business, and, with the high-rise-spiked bluffs of New Jersey just across the river, there is even a suggestion of the great bulk of the

continental United States looming up and rolling on to
the Pacific. Standing there, taking it all in, you can see
hundreds, even thousands of people and you can also see
where millions more are just out of sight. It is a place
where the big thing that is the whole world meets the
small thing that is the world of bad brains and nervous
systems. It is a seam, and a point of perspective. Looking down at the cars seeping in and out of the city on the
bridge entrances and exits, you see people sitting there
and you *know* that some of them are going to get sick.
You can imagine it happening. You can imagine the man
in the red Ford wondering why the cigarette dropped out
of his fingers, and why he didn't feel it go. You can imagine the first itch of a long illness in the scalp of the woman
in the silver station wagon, the earliest tingle of a stroke.
Standing on that balcony at the upper end of Manhattan,
looking out into the world and at the same time sensing
the special hospital at your back, you can conjure up the
cruelly random fact of neurological disease, with its
power to lift people out of the stream of things and change
their lives forever. Stepping back inside, you can confront it.

Founded in 1909, the Neurological Institute of New
York was the first hospital in the United States dedicated
solely to the treatment of disorders of the human nervous
system. Though it occupies its own building and still
sports a name that rings with independence, Neuro, as it
is called by those who work there, is in fact a part of the
Columbia Presbyterian Medical Center and has been for
years. But its physical autonomy is important and contributes to the common perception, held by patients, doctors, and staff alike, that Neuro is unique. In most
hospitals, the neurosurgery and neurology departments
simply occupy suites of offices down the hall from everything else, and they have to share beds, nurses, operating
rooms, and diagnostic equipment with all the other departments. At Neuro, neurosurgery and neurology are
the only action there is. From the basement, where the
CAT scans and angiograms are done, to the fourteenth
floor, where the library is located, there is a palpable
unity of purpose. Undiluted by the presence of other

departments, the specialties and subspecialties that make up the Neurological Institute seem even more special. It is a hospital within a hospital, a self-contained entity with its own address and its own history. There is a sense of coordination and a real sense of place, rare effects in the sprawl of a major urban medical center. When the Neuro nurses made up buttons to attract recruits from the rest of Columbia Presbyterian, the message was simple. "Get up your nerve," the buttons read, "come to Neuro."

Considered one of the top neurological hospitals in the world, Neuro attracts patients from all over. Each year some 3,600 patients pass through its 204 beds, and more than 1,500 of them undergo neurosurgery. Because of their reputations and the hospital's reputation, the neurosurgeons and neurologists at Neuro regularly get to see some of the most complicated and exotic cases in their fields. In addition, Neuro draws patients from the local population by way of the outpatient clinics and the emergency room at Columbia Presbyterian. This makes for an eclectic group; it's not unusual to find the victim of a neighborhood street fight, with no insurance or other apparent way to pay his bills, sharing the ICU with a wealthy foreigner whose money has enabled him to search the world for the best treatment available.

Because Neuro is a teaching hospital, two things are going on all the time—patients are being treated and residents are being trained. In the neurosurgery department there are ten residents, two at each level of the five-year program. They work under the guidance of a dozen staff neurosurgeons, experienced doctors known as attending physicians and referred to simply as "attendings." In the neurology department there are twenty-nine residents in a three-year program, and they work with a staff of more than fifty attending neurologists, research neurologists, and neuroscientists.

At Neuro, as is the case at most teaching hospitals, the residents—known collectively as the house staff—do most of the work. They are doctors in training, and it is their fate to get up too early in the morning and to go to bed too late at night. They are apprentices and they must live each day with the inherent paradox of that ancient role: much of the time they are either overqualified or under-qualified for the job at hand. One moment they are grumbling through some scut work that in their opinion would be better left to a lowly medical student, and the next moment they are sweating through a crisis in the ICU. Theirs is a world that is not so neatly divided into what they know and what they don't know; what they have seen and what they haven't seen; what they have done and what they haven't done. This classic tension is exacerbated by the fact that the mistakes residents make can kill people.

The first thing you notice about the young doctors who make up the house staff at Neuro is their overactive speech centers—they never shut up. They start talking when morning rounds begin and they keep on talking all through the day and into the night. They talk about things most people don't even want to think about: meningiomas, glioblastomas, Alzheimer's disease, arteriovenous malformations, strokes, multiple sclerosis, and more—all the things that can go wrong in the human nervous system and all the things they need to know to confront these failures of order.

Neuro is logical, they joke, and constant talk is a key tool in their struggle to grasp that logic and stay afloat in a sea of medical details. They talk to each other and to themselves. They talk to the nurses and to the attendings. They talk to the patients and to the patients' families. They mumble and they shout. They ask questions and they answer them. They give diagnoses and opinions. They argue and they agree. They address conferences and take phone calls. They talk in the elevators and in the ORs and out on the corner at the hot dog cart. The talk never stops, and somehow, to somebody, it is all important.

"This is the dead guy and this is what death smells like. A mix of sweat and . . . um . . . death." Morning rounds on the neurosurgery service. The dead guy got hit on the head with a baseball bat. Now he's hooked up to a respirator and shows no neurological function. He will die for real several days later. This morning, though, with sunlight splashing through the window, his chest is still moving up and down. His room is warm and close and smells slightly sour. His head is wrapped in white bandages and his eyes are partly open. Dead eyes, they glisten. The small band of residents and medical students just nod at the chief resident's observation and drift out of the room. There's nothing to be done for the dead guy; they are talking about other things.

Marion, a heavyset woman of fifty-one, is sitting up in bed, grinning. "Well, what do you think?" Her white hair has been shaved, the left side of her head is bald.

"I love it," the chief resident says. "How do you feel?"

"I think I'll start one of those punk rock bands," says Marion.

The day before, Marion's operation was explained to her. The risks were pointed out, and she was warned about the possibility of stroke, blindness, and paralysis. As she signed the form okaying the surgery, she smiled at the resident who had given her the "doom and gloom," as it is called. "Okay, Doctor," she said, "my life is in your hands."

A middle-aged man is sitting on the edge of his bed. His operation a success, he is going home to Texas. The residents, who have seen him every day of his stay, wish him luck. As he thanks them, he starts to cry.

A sixty-eight-year-old Hispanic man who has undergone a nine-hour operation for two brain aneurysms—balloonlike swellings in the walls of arteries—is lying in his bed cursing to himself. He is angry and confused because he is having a lot of trouble speaking, and he refuses to look at the residents or to respond to their questions. He doesn't realize that his mumbled curses are a good sign. Later, tests will reveal that he has suffered a slight stroke either during or since the surgery.

In the ICU the residents are gathered around a crib, discussing the case of a five-year-old boy operated on the day before. Suddenly he wakes up and cries for his mother. "She'll be here soon," he is told.

Sipping coffee, munching fruit, eating yogurt from cups and using tongue depressors for spoons, the residents walk the halls in the daily ritual of morning rounds. The patients are divided among several teams of residents and medical students, and as these small groups move from bedside to bedside reviewing the facts of each case and noting new developments, the sleepy calm of morning slowly dissolves. It is a relatively low-key time that establishes a sense of order as yet another long hospital day gets under way. Though standing in an ICU surrounded by critically ill people, many of whom have their heads swathed in white bandages, may seem like an unsettling and even disturbing way to start each day, for the Neuro residents it is simple routine, part of the job. In fact, for the neurosurgery residents the daily tour of patients is particularly mellow compared to what follows. When their rounds are finished, they head for the tenth floor, where the operating rooms are.

It is any Monday morning, or any Tuesday afternoon. It is any day on the tenth floor, and the Neuro operating rooms are all busy. In the hall, an unwatched color TV monitor displays the shining pink-and-red interior of someone's brain. An operation is being videotaped. In the middle of the TV picture the thin silver probe of the surgeon can be seen gently prodding the narrow white band that is the optic nerve. In the operating room, at the source of the picture, a resident is sitting at the microscope. He has slipped off his shoes for a moment and is barefoot. He is in the posture of microsurgery: his hands are held up and out before him like a conductor's and his head is bent down away from them as he peers into the scope. Just beyond the optic nerve he finds the blood vessel he is looking for. Peering into the large, two-man microscope, he watches the results of his tiny movements as if from a distance. An attending is at his side, also watching. As the resident begins to expose more of the blood vessel, the attending speaks. "Don't pull on that artery too hard," he says.

That brain surgeons, like carpenters and electricians, must learn their trade is not exactly a comforting thought. Ideally, one imagines, it would be otherwise; brain surgeons would spring whole into existence. They would simply appear out of nowhere, eminent, wise, clear of eye and steady of hand, packed solid with technical knowledge. Old but not too old, they would have perfect bedside manners, surpassed in perfection only by their talents in the operating room. Every operation would be a success; no patient would ever die.

Of course, brain surgeons are human, like their patients, and brain surgery is an acquired skill. Though carried out on a most fantastic field, it remains a most practical business. And the only way to learn it is to open up people's skulls and practice.

Learning to be a brain surgeon is like learning to fly planes off aircraft carriers, according to Dr. Donald Quest, forty-eight, who has done both. "That takes a lot of confidence, to do something like that, right?" says Quest, a staff surgeon at Neuro who also did his residency there. "To land a plane in the middle of the night, in the rain? Neurosurgery is a similar thing. You start out with the simplest things and you build on them, imperceptibly almost, layer by layer, to the point where you're doing really complicated stuff and you feel like you can do it, you know? You can still make a mistake. The best pilots crash once in a while. You can still have a problem in the OR, make a mistake yourself, or have something happen that you can't control, but even so, you know what you are doing, you know what's happening."

Obviously, a program based on the almost imperceptible accumulation of experience over the course of five years was not designed to exploit the unbounded self-confidence and gung-ho mentality of the average neurosurgical resident. Cutting open human heads is an inherently aggressive way to make a living, and the people who choose to do it are not the type who take well to the slow track. Brain surgeons, even nascent brain surgeons, want to do things, they want to act. It is not in their nature merely to observe. Yet that is exactly what the residents must do. For years they must stand by and watch others operate.

They do get to participate during their first two years in the OR. They cut scalps, they open skulls, and they keep the field of operation clear of blood using a low-pressure vacuum instrument called a sucker. In addition, they perform a task that, above all others, has come to

symbolize the junior resident's status as exalted by-
stander: at the operating surgeon's command they work
the floor pedal that controls the current in the electric
cautery, an instrument for cutting and cauterizing tissue.
("I once counted every tile in Room A," a surgeon says
as he recalls the pedal-pushing days of his first year at
Neuro.) But the primary function of the residents in the
early stages of their training is to see—to see and to remember. And if standing by tends to temper the young
surgeons' enthusiasm for life in the OR, then the system
is working.

"You can be technically a whiz kid, and you can be
very bright and intelligent, but a lot of things that go on
during an operation draw on one's experience," says Dr.
Bennett Stein, fifty-seven, chairman of Neuro's neurosurgery department. "I may know anatomy books cold.
I may have been in the laboratory and dissected, I may
be very skillful. But if I have not seen it before in life,
then I probably won't recognize it for what it is when I
see it in the operating room. The colors, textures, and
changes in contour are extremely important when we are
operating."

Outside the OR, the residents' training involves the
absorption of a constant stream of technical articles published in the *Journal of Neurosurgery* and the many other
arcane periodicals that constitute "the literature" (as in
the oft-heard query "Is there anything in the literature
on that?"). They must also consume mega-textbooks,
such as a two-volume, three-thousand-page work on angiograms, that are thick with a jargon so specialized it is
virtually a foreign language. Living in the shadow of this
mountain of printed matter, the residents come to speak
of "the reading" much as Sisyphus might speak of "the
rock." Every night, after ten- and twelve-hour days in
the hospital, they all go home and read. The neurosurgical residency also includes a six-month tour of duty on
the neurology service and three-month stints in neuroradiology and neuropathology. But all of this, including
a new wrinkle in the education of surgeons—watching
videotapes of operations—merely supports the work they
do in the operating room. Everything points there, and

the learning experience is informed by the genuine urgency of true-life situations. All the operations are for real; there are no dry runs.

What is most overwhelming about the life the residents lead on the tenth floor is the relentlessness of it. Any neurosurgical procedure is intense; whenever the brain is exposed, you can feel the tingle in the operating room: it doesn't get any heavier than this. But even that is magnified by the endless series of operations the residents take part in. While each attending is limited to two or three operations per week, the residents, who assist all the attendings, are in the ORs five and sometimes six and seven days a week. Depending on the procedures involved, they can participate in as many as three operations in a day.

As busy as they are, the residents are taught never to get used to performing brain surgery, never to take anything for granted. They learn that when you have seen one brain you have definitely not seen them all.

The key to a successful operation, everyone at Neuro agrees, is planning. "You have to teach an approach to a problem," says Dr. Jost Michelsen, fifty-two, "a logical approach to any problem. And the nervous system lends itself to that very well because it is a very logical, organized part of the body."

In practice, this entails long discussions among the attendings and the residents about how a specific operation is going to go, from opening to closing. Every step is planned in advance: where they have to go in the brain, how they are going to get there, what anatomical landmarks they are going to look for on the way in, what they are going to find at the location of the problem, what they are going to do about it, and how they are going to get back out again. They talk through the entire procedure; the residents may read up on it or view a tape of a similar operation.

All this is necessary because, as Stein points out, "It's easy to get lost. You focus on the details and sometimes you get carried away and you get lost in the brain. That sounds terrible but it is possible."

Stein, one of the best neurosurgeons in the country, is

unlikely to get lost in a brain. But his concern for even that remote possibility is typical. Neurosurgeons are obsessed by disaster. The things they think about when they think about an operation are the things that can go wrong, and the attendings pound this way of thinking into the residents. They are taught to imagine and to be prepared for the worst at all times. And they are the most alert for problems of their own making. As Dr. Abe Steinberger said at the end of his fifth and final year as a neurosurgical resident at Neuro, "I always think, when I'm doing a case, 'What can I do now to screw up?' "

As one of the two chief residents, Steinberger was undergoing the baptism by fire that would transform him from a bright young prospect into a full-blown operating neurosurgeon. He was operating every day under the critical eyes of the attendings, finally putting to use all the information he had absorbed during the thousands of hours he had spent assisting as a junior resident.

"In the fifth year we are in the process of honing them and smoothing them," says Stein. "We are bringing them up to the point where they can go out and work independently of us."

Technically, chief residents are learning how to function on their own deep inside the human brain. Having been exposed to as many surgical styles as there are attendings, they must now decide which techniques work best for them. As they refine their technical skills, they also learn the nuances of good surgical judgment—whom to operate on in the first place, what risks to take, what risks not to take—things that can really be understood and exercised only by the man in charge, the man doing the operation. And in their dealings with patients and families they find out about the ironies of honesty and the true nature of compassion. "You feel terrible," Steinberger said, discussing patients doomed by malignant tumors. "You never become immune to feeling miserable. If you do, you turn into a real schmuck."

Stocky, with thinning brown hair and large eyeglasses, Steinberger was garrulous even by neurosurgical-resident standards. He was something of a comedian, compulsively conducting the kind of corny running monologue

in which every joke is moderately funny and vaguely familiar—stuff one might expect to hear in the near-empty
lounge of a scruffy motel on the farthest outskirts of Las
Vegas. "I don't want to say my new girl is a dog or
anything, but I took her for a drive the other night and
she spent the whole time with her head out the window,"
went one line Steinberger delivered early one morning
on the tenth floor. Though he got a lot of his jokes from
joke books, Steinberger was also naturally funny in the
jumpy way of the class clown; and he was full of Jewish-
doctor jokes.

Steinberger, an Orthodox Jew whose father owned a
deli not far from Neuro, was perhaps the most knowl-
edgeable among his fellow residents. His mastery of the
literature was taken for granted; he was asked a lot of
questions about it, and he could reel off long lists of
articles on any neurosurgical subject with ease, giving a
synopsis of each if necessary. Looking and acting more
comfortable in his scrubs than in a shirt and tie, he loved
the technical aspects of neurosurgery, and was full of the
surgeon's pragmatism. Confronted with a brain tumor,
Steinberger's instinct was to say, "It's there—take the
damn thing out." He believed that his skills were best
put to use in the operating room, and that is where he
wants to be. "I sympathize with the patients," he said.
"I feel very bad when they're sick and I feel great when
they're better. But what I want to do is operate. I want
to get in there and do it."

As the brain surgeons arrive each morning on the tenth
floor, the first patients of the day are there on stretchers
in the hall, waiting for the anesthesiologists. Beneath thin
gowns the patients are naked and scared. It is the biggest
day of their lives. From now on there will be life before
the operation and life after the operation. Their heads are
going to be opened. They stare at the ceiling and smile
weakly when greeted. The surgeons walk past them as
they head for the coffee room.

The coffee room has three windows and a view that
everybody ignores. It has a big refrigerator for food and
a smaller one for blood. Along one wall the light-blue

scrubs that everybody wears (medium fits all but the largest and the smallest, and they are designed with double pockets so they are never inside out) are stacked on shelves that reach to the ceiling. There is a water fountain, a sink in the corner, a table with a white tablecloth, and a wheezing coffee machine that was rescued from the street and put into working order. If the operating rooms are the front lines, the coffee room is that strangely calm area just behind them where strategies are planned, time is killed, and rest is taken. It is a place of serious talk and of rambling, inconsequential conversation. It is a hangout. The brain surgeons eat their lunch there.

The brain surgeons' locker room is an equally normal place. Two large windows face west, catching the afternoon sun and affording a partial view of the Hudson River and the George Washington Bridge. It's a small room with lockers lined up along three walls. Two old leather armchairs and a huge old wooden desk take up almost half the floor space. It has about it the air of an old men's club. There are stacks of medical journals on the windowsills. A rolling hamper in the middle of the room is for scrubs, and by late afternoon it is overflowing. Every now and then a beeper will go off inside a locked locker and beep until the battery dies. The oddest thing about the locker room is the shoes. White shoes, worn and spattered with dried blood, are scattered about on the floor. Kicked off and forgotten, they lie in corners and under the desk, catching dust. Shoes for operating in are a priority for the surgeons; the operations take so long the doctors must have comfortable shoes. Some surgeons have shoes that they wear only on the tenth floor; they keep them in a special shelf in the hall. Others operate in shoes they wear in off the street, and so they must cover them with sterile booties before they go into the operating room. Old shoes are abandoned in the locker room and drift about there seemingly forever.

On a reception desk in the hall is a large book in which each operation is recorded by hand. It is a distinctly old-fashioned, leather-bound ledger that covers a year's time. Each entry lists the name of the patient, the type of procedure, the attending surgeon in charge, and the residents assisting. It is made out a day in advance, and the residents check it to learn their immediate fate—who gets to do what with whom. Reactions range from the moans of those who find themselves assigned to simple procedures or unpopular attendings to the quick claps and hoots of the ones who land rare or exciting cases.

Just inside the swinging doors that separate the working area of the tenth floor from the elevator area is the light board where the surgeons review CAT scans, angiograms, and X rays before heading into the ORs. Hung on the wall at eye level, the light board each morning draws clusters of residents and attendings into its small arc of harsh light. As "the pictures" go up, the surgeons, each with his head cocked at a different angle, once more study the jammed interiors of their patients' heads. Since as many as four operations can get under way at one time, the surgical teams overlap in front of the light board, and information and opinions are freely exchanged.

"Look at this. It's a textbook beauty." Abe Steinberger was in front of the light board studying an angiogram, in this case a radiologic map of a man's cerebral blood supply. The translucent profile of the skull is filled with a tangle of dark, wormy arteries. To the untrained eye it is incomprehensible, but Steinberger is genuinely excited by what he sees. "There," he said, pointing at the skull, "see the displacement. Tumor did that."

It was Monday morning. Directed by Stein, Steinberger was going after a large tumor compressing the brainstem of a thirty-one-year-old man. It was a rare operation, a suboccipital craniectomy, a supracerebellar infratentorial approach. That is, into the back of the head and over the cerebellum, under the tentorium to the brainstem and the tumor. Stein had done the operation more than fifty times, more than any other surgeon in the United States. Many neurosurgeons consider brainstem tumors of this type inoperable because of their location and treat them instead with radiation. "It's where you live," said Steinberger, talking about the brainstem. Literally and figuratively, it is the core of the organ. Operating on it is always risky.

As often happens in neurosurgery, the symptoms in this case did not seem to match the drastic nature of the problem. The man complained of severe headaches, nausea, and an increasingly unsteady gait. These are serious enough, but somehow they seem an inadequate way for such a terrible tumor to announce itself. Of course, the alternative—a cataclysmic event, a bolt out of the blue—is no better. And the ultimate tyranny of the disease is the same, whether it slips in the cellar window or comes crashing through the roof.

The patient lay naked and unconscious in the center of the cool, tiled room. His head was shaved, his eyes and nose taped shut. His mouth bulged with the ventilator that was breathing for him. Clear plastic tubes carried anesthetic into him and urine out of him. Belly up under the bright lights, he looked large and helpless, exposed. He was not dreaming; he was too far under for that. The depth of his obliviousness was accentuated by the urgent activity of the nurses and technicians moving in and out of the room preparing the instruments of surgery. At his head, Steinberger and the junior resident Bob Solomon stood discussing the approach they would use in the operation. As they talked, they traced possible incisions across the patient's scalp with their fingers.

The patient was then clamped into a sitting position. Before the first incision was made, he was rolled under the raised instrument table, and he disappeared beneath sterile green drapes and towels. The only part of him left exposed was the back of his head, which was orange from the sterilizing agent painted on it. Using a special marking pen, Steinberger drew the pattern of the opening on the patient's head in blue. Then the first cut was made into the scalp, and a thin line of bright-red blood appeared.

Operations take place within what is called the sterile field, a small germ-free zone created and vigilantly patrolled by the OR nurses. The sterile field extends out and around from the surgical opening and up over the instrument table. Once robed and gloved, the doctors and scrub nurses are considered sterile from the neck to

the waist and from the hands up the arms to just below
the shoulders.

Of all the rituals of surgery, the most striking is the
scrubbing of the hands. Leaning over the troughlike
stainless-steel sink with their masks in place and their
arms lathered to the elbow, the surgeons attend to each
finger with the brush and work their way up each arm in
the part of their routine that most completely cuts them
off from the rest of the world. It is a simple act raised to
sacramental heights, an obsessive, exaggerated version
of an everyday occurrence that avoids being absurd by
being so important. It is the final pause, the last thing
the surgeons do before they enter the operating room and
go to work. Many at Neuro are markedly quiet while they
scrub; they spend the familiar moments silently running
through the operation one more time. When they finish
and their hands are too clean for anything but surgery,
they turn off the water with knee controls and back
through the OR door, their dripping hands held high
before them. They dry off with sterile towels, step into
long-sleeved robes, and then plunge their hands into thin
surgical gloves, which are held out for them by the scrub
nurse. The gloves snap as the nurse releases them around
the doctors' wrists. Unnaturally smooth and defined, the
gloved hands of the neurosurgeons are now ready; they
can touch the living human brain.

The human skull is not designed for easy opening. It
takes drills and saws and simple force to breach it. It is
a formidable container, and its thickness testifies to the
value of its contents. Opening the skull is one of the first
things the residents get to do on their own. It is sometimes called cabinetwork.

"Drill the hell out of it," Steinberger said to Solomon.
The scalp had been retracted and the skull exposed. Solomon pressed the large stainless-steel power drill against
the bone and hit the trigger. The bit turned slowly, biting
into the white skull. Shavings dropped from the hole onto
the drape and then to the floor. The drill stopped automatically when it was through the bone. The hole was
about a half-inch in diameter. Solomon drilled four holes
in a diamond pattern. The skull at the back of the head

was ridged and bumpy. There was a faint odor of burning bone.

The drilling was graphic and jarring. The drill and the head did not go together; they collided and shocked the eye. The tool was too big, its scale and shape inappropriate to the delicate idea of neurosurgery. It should have been hanging on the wall of a garage. After the power drill, a hand drill was used to refine the holes in the skull. It was a sterilized stainless-steel version of a handyman's tool. It was called a perforator, and as Solomon calmly turned it, more shavings hit the floor. Then, using powerful plierlike tools called rongeurs, the surgeons bit away at the skull, snapping and crunching bone to turn the four small holes into a single opening about three inches in diameter. This was a craniectomy; the hole in the skull would always be there, protected by the many layers of scalp muscle at the back of the head. The other technique for opening a skull is a craniotomy, in which a flap of bone is preserved to cover the opening in the skull.

After the scalp and the skull, the next layer protecting the brain is the dura mater. A thin, tough, leathery membrane that encases the brain, the dura (derived from the Latin word for *hard*) is dark pink, almost red. It is rich with blood vessels and nerves (when you have a headache, it's the dura that aches), and now it could be seen stretching across the expanse of the opening, pulsing lightly. The outline of the cerebellum bulging against the dura was clear. With a crease in the middle, the dura-sheathed cerebellum looked oddly like a tiny pair of buttocks. The resemblance prompted a moment's joking. "Her firm young cerebellum," somebody said.

Because the patient was in a sitting position, there was a constant danger of air getting into the bloodstream, and so a monitor that amplified the sound of the blood flowing through the heart was in place. The sound of the whoosh and rush of the pumping blood filled the operating room. It had a deep gurgling rhythm of its own, and as the dura was being opened, that rhythm was suddenly broken by a higher, racketing sound; a tiny bubble of air was in the bloodstream. Steinberger quickly jammed the hole in the head with surgical sponges as the anesthesiologist adjusted his equipment and coolly reported to Steinberger at the same time. It was a life-threatening emergency, but it was quickly brought under control, and gradually the sound of the beating heart returned to normal.

The dura was then carefully opened and sewn back out of the way. An hour and fifteen minutes after the drilling began, the brain was exposed.

The brain exposed. It happens every day at Neuro, three, four, and five times a day, day after day, week in and week out, month after month. The brain exposed. Light falls on its gleaming surface for the first time. It beats lightly, steadily. It is pink and gray, the brain, and covered with tiny blood vessels, in a web. In some openings you can see the curve of the brain, its roundness. It does not look strong, it looks very soft, soft enough for you to push your finger through. When you see it for the first time, you almost expect sparks arcing across the surface of the cortex, blinking lights, the crackle of an idea. You stare down at it, and it gives nothing back, reveals nothing, gives no hint of how it works. It is the glistening pulp at the center of everything, and as soon as surgeons see it, they begin the search for landmarks. They start talking to each other, describing what they both can see, narrating the anatomy.

In the operating room the eyes bear much of the burden of communication. With their surgical masks and caps in place, the doctors and nurses resort to exaggerated stares and squints and flying eyebrows to emphasize what they are saying and to respond to what others say. After more than three decades in the operating room, Dr. Stein has developed this talent to a fine art. His eyes narrowed in concentration as he listened to Steinberger explain what he wanted to do next. They discussed how to go about retracting the cerebellum. "Okay, Abe," Stein said quietly. "Nice and easy now."

The cerebellum (the word means "little brain") is one of the most complicated parts of the brain. It is involved in the processing of sensory information of all kinds as well as balance and motor control, but in this case it was simply in the way. With the dura gone the cerebellum bulged out of the back of the head; it could be seen from across the room, protruding into space, striated and strange-looking.

When the cerebellum was retracted, a two-man microscope with a cable running to a TV monitor and a videotape machine was rolled into place. Sitting side by side, looking through the scope into the head, Steinberger and Stein started searching for the tumor.

The development of the operating microscope has had a major impact on all aspects of neurosurgery. Not only has it enabled today's brain surgeons to see things they couldn't twenty-five years ago, it has transformed the training process. Now the resident and attending can share one pair of eyes; they can enter the brain together, see the same things at the same time. As a result, the residents get to do more. "It's easier to give them hands-on experience," says Stein. "With the microscope you can control the operation as the teacher."

It is a long and tedious process, working your way into the center of the human brain. The joke about the slip of the scalpel that wiped out fifteen years of piano lessons is no joke. Every seen and unseen piece of tissue does something, has some function, though it may well be a mystery to the surgeon. The neurons are linked up in ways beyond current understanding, and so any cut or burn is potentially damaging. "When you first start operating," Steinberger says, "every time you touch the brain you say, 'Oh my God, what if this is an important part?'" That mix of fear and respect is one reason neurosurgical procedures take as long as they do. Things that are technically simple, like taking out a tumor, are rendered complex by the location. It's like changing your pants on the wing of an airplane in flight. Changing your pants is no big deal, but where you do it makes all the difference. (For the analogy to be complete, though, someone else would have to plunge to his death if you slipped.) As Stein points out, "It's true that getting out the interior of a tumor with curettes or scoops or suction is not very elegant. But it's a matter of having a concept of where everything is located, three dimensions. Then, when you start to work around the margin of the tumor, it's not like a piece of intestine that you can sort of bat aside, and hack off if it bleeds. All the little details of anatomy have to be sorted out.''

After two hours of talking and dissecting their way through the glowing red geography of the inner brain, Stein and Steinberger came upon the tumor. ''Holy Toledo, look at that,'' exclaimed Steinberger. The tumor stood out from the tissue around it, purple and mean-looking. It was the end of order in a very small, orderly place. It did not belong. Sitting there in the middle of the sterile field, in the center of nature's most refined bundle of cells, the tumor was a shock and a contradiction. They paused a moment, and Steinberger gave a quick tour of the opening. ''That's tumor, that's the brainstem, and that's the third ventricle,'' he said, pointing. ''And that over there, that's memory.''

Basically, every brain operation consists of three parts—getting to the location of the problem, treating the problem, and getting back out again. Getting in and getting out, simple matters in most other kinds of surgery, become important in neurosurgery because, as Stein notes, there are no unimportant parts of the brain. Even so, there is a different tone to the operation during these bookend stages. During the approach there is a lighter feel to things in the OR, brought on in part by the pleasure surgeons like Stein take in seeing the anatomy, touring around in the brain, and enjoying the sights. At the end of the operation, there is an understandable easing of tension as they back out and close up the head. But in between, there is a time when it is all on the line. It may be a period of seconds or minutes or even hours. It is the surgical moment, the heart of the operation, when the risks are greatest and the concentration is deepest as the surgeon at last confronts the disease, his hands deep in the patient's head, the red hole shining under the OR lights, as though lit from within. Everything leads up to it, and then it all leads away from it.

Over the course of two hours, with Stein watching his every move, Steinberger carefully took the tumor. (Brain surgeons ''take'' tumors and, when necessary, they ''take'' brain.) When he used the cautery to burn out pieces of the deadly tissue, smoke rose from the hole in the head in a faint, twisting wisp. At one point, Stein unpacked his camera and took a picture for his records. Using a special lens he leaned in and snapped away, excited by the rare and vivid view of the brainstem. A doctor from the pathology department showed up for a piece of the tumor and carried it away in a small plastic cup. It was analyzed while the operation was still under way so the surgeons could know what they were dealing with. The type of tumor plays an important part in decisions about how much to take out and what risks to take in an attempt to get it all. Getting the whole tumor is called, appropriately, gross total removal.

This tumor turned out to be a brainstem glioma, an invasive, intrinsic tumor actually growing up out of the brainstem. It was malignant. They got a lot of it but they could not get it all and it would grow back. With radiation treatment the patient could live fifteen years or so, and he would be told so. Abe Steinberger would tell him.

As he was closing, Steinberger was asked if he thought he had helped the patient. "Now we know what it is," he said, meaning the exact pathology of the tumor. "And we took a lot of it." The bottom line is, he added, that the results of the surgery should be at least equal to the results of no surgery; if you can decompress and identify the tumor without making the patient worse than he was before the surgery, then you have helped the patient.

During the closing, Steinberger had a bit of trouble cauterizing a tiny blood vessel near the surface of the opening, what the surgeons call a "bleeder." "You gotta make sure it's dry before you leave," he said as he finally stopped the trickle of blood. More than six hours after the first incision, the operation ended.

When the surgery was over, a new anxiety came into play as the surgical team waited to see if the patient would wake. As the anesthesiologist slowly brought the patient "up," the surgeons stood around the operating table watching for signs of consciousness. In this particular case, because of where they were working, there was extra concern for the patient's post-op condition; operating on and near major structures like the brainstem and the cerebellum can leave people comatose, or with serious neurological deficits.

"Hey, George! Wake up, George!" the anesthesiologist called loudly. Taking the patient's hand, Steinberger called to him as well. "Squeeze my hand, Mr. Thomas. Come on, squeeze my hand!" Out from under the drapes now, the patient was a man again, no longer just a small red hole in the middle of a field of green. His head was wrapped in a turban of white bandages. Gradually he emerged from immobile unconsciousness into a kind of troubled sleep. He moaned lightly and moved his head. This pleased the doctors and they urged him on. "Come on, George, move your legs. Can you move your legs?" "Open your eyes, Mr. Thomas." The immediate post-op exam is a primitive and disturbing thing: Can you see? Can you hear? Can you feel this? In neurosurgery, even "successful" operations can leave patients with serious deficits. Eventually George came up enough to satisfy the doctors; he moved all his limbs. He was then transferred to a hospital bed and wheeled out of the OR to the elevator and taken down to the ICU on the ninth floor.

The next day, Steinberger's automatic resident's fear of screwing up the case went unrealized when George Thomas woke up fresh.

"The thing about neurosurgery which is different from other surgeries," says Bennett Stein, "is the tremendous variety of operations. We're operating on every part of the body; on the extremities for nerves, on the back, the spinal column, the brain. We use all sorts of routes; through the ear, through the mouth, through the belly or the chest to get to the front part of the spine. You don't get blasé about any of these because they are all a little bit different."

Stein estimates that in the twenty-four years since he completed his residency at Neuro he has performed nearly 4,500 operations, at the rate of 150 to 200 per year. As is the case with most modern neurosurgeons, Stein has several operations that he specializes in. He is best known as a vascular neurosurgeon. When it comes to removing arteriovenous malformations—clusters of excess blood vessels—in the brain or spinal cord, he is at the top of his field. He also has a few other "series" going, operations he does more of than most other neurosurgeons, like the brainstem glioma.

Stein has sharp blue eyes and an easy smile. He is in good physical condition, medium in height with the solid shoulders and the square build of a middleweight. Though he is outwardly calm and easygoing, it is not difficult to detect his underlying sense of determination and his faith in himself and his judgments. And he is as sure of himself behind his desk as he is in the OR or at a patient's bedside in the ICU. After more than fifteen years as a department chief, first at Tufts and now at Neuro, Stein knows his way around the ego-clogged halls of big-time medicine as well as he does around the brain. Running things seems to come naturally to him. As he notes with a laugh when discussing the various surgical styles the residents are exposed to and must choose from, "But you see the dilemma that the residents have, and they know it, is that when they are working with me they do it my way."

Though he has mastered the administrative and academic aspects of his specialty as well as anyone could and has landed one of the plum jobs in a very competitive field, Stein has not availed himself of the opportunity to become a bastard. Tradition allows for chiefs of surgery to carry on like despots, but that fashion is fading. Indeed, though Stein likes to see things done his way in the OR, since he took over at Neuro in late 1980, the residents have been able to do more and do it sooner than ever before. "This place has changed incredibly," said Abe Steinberger, whose first four years were very traditional and, for him, very frustrating. "There's before Stein and after Stein," he said, "and they are completely different eras."

Stein's career as a brain surgeon stretches from 1960, when he began his residency, and covers what is without doubt the period of greatest advancement in the field since the first thirty years of this century, when Harvey Cushing was blazing his way through those primitive ORs. When Stein was starting out, there was no CAT scan and the microscope was only just coming into use. "There were operations when we weren't exactly sure what we were going to find or exactly where it was," recalls Stein. "And sometimes we'd end up off the area or we'd open up and find everything was absolutely normal. Now you just don't get those errors because of the absolute certainty of what we're operating on, because of the sophistication of the diagnostic workup."

Not everything about those days was bad. Like other surgeons who worked in the years before the CAT scan, Stein has good memories of some of the old techniques. "What's fallen by the wayside in our field is the old classic diagnosis, the fun of it. Sitting down with the old neurological exam and spending an hour checking this, checking that, interviewing the patient. Like a gourmet meal, sitting there and enjoying every course of it, and then coming up with a diagnosis. Now it's a quick exam, get a scan and an arteriogram."

What Stein enjoys more than anything is operating. He is enamored of the nervous system, of neuroanatomy. He loves seeing the brain and working on it. "The thing about the nervous system that I think is truly different from any other specialty system or organ system in the body is that it's very well arranged," says Stein. "It's like an electrical diagram, it's an electrical engineer's dream." In fact, Stein had originally planned to be an engineer, like his father. "I sort of had that engineering type of mind." But he chose medicine and then, while in his first year at the Dartmouth medical school, he took a course in neuroanatomy. It left him "completely befuddled." "It can be extremely detailed or extremely logical, depending on the way it's presented," Stein explains. "If you learn the logic of it, it becomes easy because the details then all fall into place. But if you try to learn it from the details side, then you're lost. And that's the way it was being taught and I abhorred that."

Then, in his second year of medical school, Stein was exposed to a neurosurgeon in the clinic at Dartmouth, and the lights came on. "All of a sudden this course which had been a dismal part of my life became exciting. Neuroanatomy made sense, you could see it applied to the patients. And I liked things that made sense, that came together in a logical way.''

Stein loves microsurgery. ''It's anatomical, it's beautiful,'' he says, rhapsodizing about the way the brain looks through the scope. ''We look upon, say, cardiac or general surgery as being very gross,'' says Stein, emphasizing the word *gross*. ''Your hands are in there and you're pushing things around. And here we're working with little instruments, and the critics say, 'Well, you're diddling around in a space the size of a quarter for hour after hour and what do you want to spend your life doing that for? That's crazy!' But brain surgery is for the individual that's fascinated by this meticulous, compulsive working in a small area.''

Though they share the human nervous system, neurosurgery and neurology are fundamentally different. It starts with the basic difference between surgical medicine and nonsurgical medicine, between invasive and noninvasive procedures. Surgeons of any specialty routinely take the most radical step available—they cut open the body and remove or repair the thing that is causing the problem. Doctors who are not surgeons remain outside the body. Using physical exams, blood tests, X rays, and other diagnostic methods, they probe the body and, in a sense, they do enter it. But their patients remain intact, and their work is primarily a matter of deduction. Though their treatment is direct—administering drugs, prescribing changes in diet and physical activity—it is not nearly as direct as the acute intervention of the surgeon. In short, there are those who cut and those who don't.

In the case of neurosurgery and neurology, the contrast is sharpened by two factors unique to neurological medicine. First, the bloody reality of surgery in general is exaggerated in neurosurgery because very often it is the head that is cut open and the brain that is operated on. This casts the neurosurgeon's job in a more graphic light. Second, neurology is a specialty with more than its share of incurable diseases, including Alzheimer's, ALS, and multiple sclerosis, to name but three. So, not only must the neurologists at Neuro work alongside the most invasive surgeons of all, they have to deal with problems that often deny them the doctor's greatest pleasure—curing the patient. The fact is, then, neurosurgeons and neurologists are at opposite extremes: while one can usually provide the most direct treatment possible, the other often can provide no treatment at all.

Which is not to say that the neurologists at Neuro are any less aggressive than their surgical colleagues. They don't drill holes in people's skulls, but they do take on some mighty nasty diseases and care for some very sick people. Not for them the daily gestalt of the OR, the completed act, the operation that begins and ends; their haul is a long one, their chief weapon not the knife but the mind. They don't get to cut, they have to think all the time. And look, and see. And, of course, talk.

"Let's talk about one confusing thing at a time." It is 9:00 A.M., and Dr. Lewis P. Rowland, sixty-three, the chief of neurology at Neuro, is presiding over "Rowland's meeting," a short conference that takes place each weekday morning in the library. With Rowland, ranged around three large tables pushed together to form a long-stemmed T, are the chief resident, a couple of attendings, and the second-year residents who head up the teams that are responsible for the daily care of the neurology patients. The first set of morning rounds is over, and the business at hand is to record new admissions and discharges, to update Rowland on the progress of particular cases, and to generally organize the daily activities of the department. Each year, some two thousand patients are admitted to the neurology service, and each of them is discussed at Rowland's meetings. Each also receives an entry in Rowland's log, a small record book in which he keeps track of every patient with cryptic notes in his own hand.

The four team leaders carry index cards of different colors on which they keep track of their patients, and they refer to these as they report to Rowland each day. There are usually about 160 neurology patients in house, and, given the complexity of the diseases involved, the information that has to be dealt with at Rowland's meeting each day can seem overwhelming. But Rowland is a relaxed, orderly man, and he keeps the details flowing smoothly. His request to limit the conversation to a single confusing topic follows an exchange in which a resident, in response to a question about a current case, refers to some research recently reported in the literature that he thinks might apply. Rowland isn't so sure it does, and he deftly splits the appropriate hair, which concerns two different conditions—myasthenia gravis, a neuromuscular disorder, and hyperthyroidism.

Though the subjects covered during Rowland's meetings are serious, the tone is usually informal. Sitting on the fourteenth floor, literally atop a heap of cases, the doctors offer each other opinions and ideas in an open forum that is remarkably free of tension and self-interest. This openness is a result of Rowland's easygoing personal style and his basic trust in the residents. "These are mature people, and if you stay out of their way they will learn what they have to learn," he says. "That has dominated my theory on teaching medical students and house staff forever. I think we have a bunch of terrific residents, and if we just leave them alone they will do what they have to do. And the system works out."

In fact, Rowland's meetings provide him with daily, direct contact with the residents, and he makes the most of it; he doesn't leave them alone, he teaches them neurology. It is the oldest of teaching methods, a modified Socratic method in which the point is not to embarrass a resident or prove him wrong but to lead him to the correct conclusion. As the residents present the facts of each case, Rowland listens and calmly questions them about their diagnoses and treatment plans. With more than thirty years as a neurologist behind him, Rowland is a certified heavyweight in the field. His credentials include a stint as the president of the American Neurological Association and an international reputation as a clinical researcher, specializing in neuromuscular disorders. He is a resource for the residents, his vast experience as valuable to them as their own. In small moments each morning, they tap into his store of knowledge and draw a little off. He takes what they tell him, chews on it, and feeds it back to them in a question or a suggestion, slightly altered, often with a new idea in it. Sometimes he doesn't say anything, he just writes in his book. Other times, with just a word or two, he will overturn a diagnosis and send the resident back for more information. Usually there is give and take as Rowland tests the residents' reasoning and forces them to defend their positions. And slowly, over time, what Rowland knows is dripped into the residents.

The cases range from the common to the rare—one year there were 362 cases of stroke admitted and four cases of Creutzfeldt-Jakob disease, a mysterious type of dementia—and each day seems to have its star case. "What a day for the social aspects of medicine," Rowland remarks one morning as a resident explains two problem cases. One involves a patient with AIDS and the other a patient who is a Jehovah's Witness and refuses blood transfusions. Another day, the hot case is a man in his thirties with an inflammatory mass in his brain that turns out to be a parasite, a neurological complication of a case of trichinosis. Yet another day, a stroke case triggers a discussion of what exactly the word *stroke* means. Some uses the term *CVA*, meaning "cerebrovascular accident," while reporting on a case, and Rowland jumps on it. He doesn't like the term. "It implies that it can be avoided if you're careful," he says, "like an automobile accident." It is a perfect example of the neurologist's mind at work, pondering the nuances of the specialty's most common language, an issue one would assume had been settled years ago. "Neurologists are supposed to be stamp collectors," Rowland explains later. "They like to classify, pigeon-hole, separate. They're neat and compulsive. But on the other hand, because they get interested in the brain and the mind, they also like to think globally." When Rowland's meeting ends, everybody heads for the elevators. The day's second set of rounds now begins. Each accompanied by an attending, the resident teams get down to the business of clinical neurology.

Second-year neurology resident Linda Kaplan headed

a team that consisted of herself, three first-year residents, and a couple of medical students who were doing a rotation through the service. The first-year residents were responsible for the day-to-day care of the team's patients. They reported to Kaplan, whose job was to oversee their work, teaching them and assisting them in the details of patient care. Watching over Kaplan and her team was an attending physician. In addition, many of the team's patients had been admitted by various staff neurologists, who also guided the team's work.

Kaplan's team was responsible for thirty-five patients, and she kept the index cards for all of them on a ring, flipping quickly to the appropriate one as each case was dealt with. Kaplan's list that day included eleven stroke patients, six patients with tumors, five with neurovascular disorders, three with Parkinson's disease, and one case each of dementia, myasthenia gravis, meningitis, encephalitis, ALS, coma, Creutzfeldt-Jakob disease, and peripheral neuropathy. Her youngest charge was a twenty-three-year-old man with a cancerous tumor of the spine; her oldest was a ninety-year-old woman with a stroke. By any measure it was an impressive collection of cases, covering virtually the entire human nervous system—and it was typical of Neuro.

"You have to do the hardest residency," said Kaplan. "You have to see the most patients. I can't believe I'm saying this, it's just the thing everybody complains about, but you have to see a lot of patients. That's how you learn, by seeing and taking care of a lot of sick people. And you only have a few years to do it, so you have to do a lot of it."

Kaplan looked several years younger than her age, thirty-one, and she had a high, sweet voice that could be described as girlish but for the fact that there was a serious edge on it much of the time, a small thing at the top end that gave her a firmer tone. Only when she was off duty or when she was dealing with patients, particularly her older, female patients, did she relax and let the natural, easy ring in her voice come through. The fact that she was an attractive young woman used to affect the way she presented herself. When she was a medical student, she used to dress in a way that she thought made her appear "older and not too frivolous." Then, as she learned her job, she stopped worrying about it. "It gets to the point where I'm going to be taking good care of this person and they're going to know it," she said. "As soon as you examine someone, you establish a relationship, and by the end of an exam I never had a patient who felt that I was anything less than fully competent."

Though she seemed unaware of it, Kaplan had the kind of face that readily reflected her feelings. Unlike doctors who have mastered the limited variety of traditional clinician faces—the all-purpose stone face, the small mirthless smile, the interested eyebrows and pursed lips—when Kaplan was tired, or angry, or pleased, when she was working out a problem or being the boss, it was all there to be seen in her animated features. And whatever her mood or the situation might be, beneath everything you could always detect a hard intelligence and a sense of determination. She was the kind of person who could say "I really like infectious disease," and you knew that she did and you knew what she meant. For Kaplan, neurology was not a morbid field but an exciting one. Incurable diseases didn't get her down, they challenged her.

"If you just look at it as a specialty where you want to make a diagnosis and make a treatment and take your money and send the patient home, then it's very boring and very depressing," Kaplan said. "You have to look at it as a research area. Because if you think about all the things you're going to discover, or the cures you're going to find, then it's exciting." In fact, many of the neurology residents at Neuro, like Kaplan, pursue careers in research. Which is not surprising, given the nature of the specialty—if your house was always burning down, you would probably give some serious thought to becoming a fireman.

Life in a hospital is different, feverish, broken off from the outside world. One measure of just how different life is in hospitals is the way things from regular life are transformed in their hospital incarnation. Beds, for instance. Outside a hospital a bed is a place of rest, where you lie down tired and get up refreshed. It's a stopping place, a temporary thing. In hospitals, if you're a patient, a bed is where you live. You eat in it and excrete in it. You are either lying in it or sitting near it. Your room is just big enough to hold it and a few other pieces of furniture and nothing more. You run your life from it. You receive guests in it. And those guests are themselves transformed by their presence in a hospital. Your friends and relatives are sucked out of their lives just as you are sucked out of yours. Into the foreign world of the hospital they are forced to come, skin crawling at the smell of medicinal alcohol and the sight of needles, drawing back from patients being wheeled down the hall or, worse, patients shuffling along under their own power in pajamas, bathrobes, and slippers, pushing their IV racks with them as they go. No visitor is comfortable in a hospital, except those visiting the maternity ward. Smiles don't mean what they usually mean, conversations are stilted.

Television is different in the hospital too. It's on constantly, from the first thing in the morning until the last thing at night. You hear it as you move down the halls, all the TVs in all the rooms, some in harmony and some tuned to different channels. The daytime lineup of game shows and soap operas lends a manic, morbid air to hospital afternoons, as one show follows another and the meaninglessness of it all piles up. What should be an escape becomes inescapable, a classic hospital transformation.

Time too is transformed in the hospital. The day starts too early in the morning and ends too early in the evening. The patients do nothing, and doctors come in and tell them they are "doing great." Lifted out of the normal world, the patient's life, usually a balanced mix of the physical and the mental, suddenly becomes skewed. The physical goes wrong, and there is new pressure on the mental to figure it all out. You are sick and you must lie there and think about that fact.

Hospitals, of course, are the doctors' turf. For the patient, it's another transformation. Here is this person, this doctor, whom you normally see once a year or so, whom you may not like all that much to begin with, and now you see him every day and his power over you is complete. The doctors are the healthy ones. They don't wear pajamas and they get to go home at night. They aren't missing work, they're at work. The patient often doesn't know what's really going on and the doctor often does.

The neurology resident teams roam Neuro in packs. Down the hall they come in their white pants, white skirts, white coats, with their laminated ID cards clipped to their shirts, their beepers on their belts, and their stethoscopes poking out of their pockets and dangling around their necks. (The beepers provide a kind of electronic theme song throughout the day. They are always going off and sending residents in search of a phone. Hospitals are the only places where people actually use the phones in elevators.) During the first set of rounds in the morning the teams visit all their patients briefly to see how the night has gone for them and how they are making out as the day begins. Then, during attending rounds, they return to a few cases that have been selected because they present particular problems. After attending rounds the teams break up, and the residents go about the endless business of moving their patients through the medical system. They talk with them, review their medication schedules, and, if necessary, adjust them. They take them to the basement for radiologic treatment. Four afternoons a week there is a neurology clinic for outpatients. They are almost absurdly busy sessions; one year, more than ten thousand patients visited. There are several special clinics, including ones for stroke, movement disorders, and neuro-oncology (cancer of the nervous system) patients. Then, in the late afternoon, the teams make yet another set of rounds.

Each night of the week there are two neurology residents and two neurosurgery residents on call in the hospital. They stay in a dorm on the first floor that recalls a small men's college circa 1929, when the Neuro building was completed. A dozen small, single rooms line a narrow hallway. Each room has a single bed, a sink, a phone by the bed, a desk, and a closet. Two to three residents are assigned to each room. They are funky spaces, cluttered with well-thumbed medical journals, worn-out stethoscope pieces, old X rays, and many pairs of white pants. At one end of the hall there is a single, white-tiled bathroom that serves all. In the residents' lounge is an old TV set, some bookshelves holding a few old volumes of the Harvard Classics, and a scattering of magazines. There are a few framed group portraits of past residents hanging on the walls and many more stacked about in careless, dusty piles.

The tradition of the overworked resident persists at Neuro; it's the price that has to be paid. The worst thing that can come of it, Linda Kaplan noted, is the doctor who resents his patients. "In the emergency room, when it's two in the morning and you've seen twelve patients and you just can't think anymore and you have no beds . . . There are times when you just feel at wit's end," she said. "I mean, you're almost, almost, put upon. The typical expression people use is 'They're hurting me'—you know, as if the doctor is hurting. It's a very egocentric way of looking at things. I've never felt that as a neurologist, but at two or three in the morning, when I get called for another patient . . . it's hard, it's hard."

Beyond the short tempers and other surface tensions created by the long, intense hours of the resident's day, another, more subtle kind of strain exists, and Kaplan described that as well. "The other day when I was on call, Sunday, I had seen this movie on the destruction of the world, called *Testament*. It is devastating. I went to a screening and I didn't know what the movie was about except in the back of my mind I remembered that there was a reason why I never wanted to see it. And I went to see the movie and came into work the next day and that morning I heard that thirty-five or forty-four Marines had been killed. Then I heard seventy-six and then some nurse comes in and says, 'Oh, a hundred and twenty-six.' And then I was called to the emergency room to see this sixty-eight-year-old German-Jewish refugee who was walking in the park and had been hit on the head with a rock and raped. And it was like 'I just don't want to hear any more, I don't want any more patients to come.' By two o'clock I had seen twelve patients. With strokes, with head trauma, with gunshot wounds. At two in the morning I was able to come back to the room and at three I got called for another patient. And it wasn't a matter of 'They're hurting me.' It was a matter of there is so much pain in the world, there is so much pain in the world, and why am I getting to see so much of it?''

At the other end of the hall from the on-call rooms is another of Neuro's collegiate elements, Zabriskie Auditorium. It is a small lecture hall that, like the dorm, harks back to the thirties. Two big wooden doors with translucent glass panels and the words ZABRISKIE AUDITORIUM painted on them open on an old hall with a low stage that has been updated with the installation of wall-hung TV monitors attached to VCRs, a modern podium, and a system of sliding blackboards and movie screens. And of course there are light boards, portable ones, for viewing X rays and CAT scans and angiograms. About 150 folding chairs have been set up so they create a center aisle, and during Grand Rounds, a regular conference that everyone attends, the attendings inevitably wind up sitting on the left side of the room and the residents on the right. On the walls of the hall hang huge oil paintings of stern-looking men, portraits of long-gone big-timers. The phone in the back of the room doesn't ring but has a light attached to it, and there is another light high on the front wall; they blink when there is a call. This is presumably designed to prevent noisy interruptions, a purpose that is defeated by the beepers. When the doctors assemble in numbers, the constant beeping is like the sound of tiny electronic frogs in random concert. No matter what the topic or how exalted the guest speaker, there is a steady shuffling to the phone and back.

In Zabriskie, the clinical and the academic elements of medical education come together in daily conferences that cover the entire range of modern neurological medicine. Grand Rounds are held weekly by both the neurosurgery service and the neurology service. (Neurosurgery Grand Rounds are sometimes taken up with what is called ''Morbidity and Mortality,'' a review of postoperative deficits and deaths.) Other regular weekly sessions include neuro-oncology, movement disorders, and neuroradiology. The information exchanged at these meetings is world class. The subjects dealt with constitute the true weight of the field. Neuro's place in the greater worlds of neurosurgery and neurology is on display in Zabriskie, where lecturers from all over the United States, Europe, and the Far East appear regularly. But the image that comes to mind, the one that best locates the old lecture hall in the larger scheme of things neurological, is that of a worn-out resident quietly dozing through a film being presented by a world-famous Japanese neurologist; as the great man's patients lurch back and forth across the screen demonstrating the severity of their movement disorders, the resident twitches in his seat, his head bowed, his fevered brain quivering in the shallows of stolen sleep.

There are plenty of graphic displays to be seen in Zabriskie. There are videotapes of operations and slide shows featuring giant, color close-ups of bloody, evil-looking tumors freshly removed from people's brains and spinal cords. But by far the most wrenching sight to be encountered there is the patients who are brought down so their cases can be presented to the doctors.

The patient waits at the back of the room while his medical history and the details of his case are laid out. Then he is wheeled to the front of the room by a resident and examined by the doctor in charge. The examinations are brief—the point is to elicit specific symptoms quickly and clearly. Patients with movement disorders are asked to rise and take a few steps. Patients with disorders of the higher cortical functions—memory or speech problems, for instance—are asked questions that reveal their condition. Most of the patients manage to retain their dignity through simple willpower—looking straight out at the doctors, making eye contact as much as possible, and maybe smiling slightly as the discussion of their case continues around them.

During these sessions the three basic elements that make up all medicine are most clearly on display: the patient, the doctor, and the disease. All the complexities of modern medicine, and everything that happens in hospitals, can be traced back to them. Every day in Zabriskie Auditorium, with the doors closed for a while against the routine chaos, the doctors and patients of Neuro pursue that kind of clarity. And in scenes stunningly vivid and human, they confront the fact that two against one isn't always such great odds.

It was a Friday night and second-year neurology resident Mitch Rubin was on night call. At 5:30 P.M., he was beeped and told there were two gunshot wounds to the head in the Columbia Presbyterian emergency room. (Neuro does not have its own E.R.) Protocol required that the neurology resident check the case out before the neurosurgery residents were brought in. As he left Neuro and walked down 168th Street, Rubin was not very excited about the gunshots. They were not good neurology, there was nothing subtle about them, and they would almost certainly be taken over by the surgeons. Calmly, Rubin strolled into the crash room, the part of the emergency suite set up for the most serious cases.

The unknown male and the unknown female lay side by side with bullet holes in their heads. The male had two holes in his head—his bullet had entered his right temple and exited the left. The female had a single hole in her head, behind her left ear. Her bullet was still buried in her brain. She also had a bullet in her chest. Rubin stepped through the crowd of emergency-room doctors and nurses surrounding the patients. Someone asked him who he was. "Neurology," he said.

The female was in worse shape than the male. She was posturing, her body stiffening in a way that signaled severe and increasing pressure on her brainstem. Her brain was swelling inside her skull and forcing her brainstem down into the foramen magnum, the hole at the base of the skull through which the brain and spinal cord connect.

For someone who had been shot in the head the male was not doing badly. He was unconscious but stable. Rubin examined both patients as well as he could, checking their eyes and some of their reflexes. As he worked, other ER staff cut off clothing and took blood samples. IVs and catheters were run as the patients were prepared for X rays. A detective in a plaid sport coat stood just outside

the crash room, notebook in hand. A uniformed police-
man was also present. It was an apparent case of attempted homicide/suicide. The pattern of the wounds
indicated that the male did the shooting. Curious residents and medical students came by to see what was going on. It was a jarring emergency case, even by New
York City standards.

In the course of taking X rays the room was cleared
and the unconscious pair was left alone. The view through
the doors of the crash room was grim and compelling.
The patients, in their twenties, looked young and healthy
but for the small, oozing wounds in their heads. They
were Hispanic, and their light-brown skin appeared soft
under the bright lights. The eerie fact was they made a
nice-looking couple. A medical student looking on was
quietly shaken by what he saw. "What a waste of life,"
he said softly. Then he turned and walked away.

Henry Brem and Bob Solomon, the neurosurgery residents on call, arrived, and it was their show now. They
checked the patients and the X rays. On the light board,
the bullet and bone fragments in the brains showed up
white inside the ghostly X-ray skulls. The decision was
made to prepare the male for surgery and to wait on the
female; she was probably beyond saving. Brem and Solomon headed back to Neuro to prepare for the operation.
They had to track down and consult with the attendings
on call and get things ready on the tenth floor. Rubin's
job was to get the patient over to Neuro, get him CAT-
scanned, and get him to the OR.

Rubin, assisted by two medical students, rolled the
gurney through the emergency suite and down the hall to
an elevator. One of the medical students was bagging the
patient—aiding his breathing by squeezing a rubber bladder over and over again, pumping air into his lungs. They
were in the public part of the hospital. Visitors waiting
near the elevators stepped back as the patient was rolled
up. Others found themselves pressed back against the wall
of an elevator as Rubin commandeered one and took it
to the basement. The gruesomeness of the wounds, earlier mitigated by the rites of the emergency room, came
back in the confines of the crowded elevator. On each

side of the patient's head the bullet holes, lightly leaking bright-red blood, formed the center of ugly, purple lumps, swollen to the size of eggs. Some people in the elevator chose to ignore the sight; others stared.

Then Rubin and his group were out of the elevator, alone and moving quickly through the creepy maze of long, narrow tunnels connecting the medical center's buildings. Steering the gurney was hard work. It was heavy and it had to be held back on a long downslope and then pushed up the other side. At one point, a doctor coming the other way had to squeeze back against the wall to let it pass. Little was said; the squeaking of the gurney wheels and the regular hiss of the air bag were the only sounds.

Arriving at the CAT scanner, Rubin's charge created another small scene of shock and fascination, this time among the technicians. The weird symmetry of the bullet holes and the calm look on the face of the man who had wanted to die combined to create a bizarre portrait of mayhem in repose. There was craziness in the air. As the patient was slipped into the scanner, a bad joke was told about a man who found another man in bed with his wife. Someone wondered if the double shooting would make the tabloids. "No," said a technician with the confidence of one who knows, "this isn't strange enough for the *Post*." When the patient was removed from the scanner, he left a smear of blood in the center of the machine.

By now Mitch Rubin was eager to be finished with the gunshot case. It was nearly seven, and he had learned that there were a couple of cases waiting for him, at least one of which sounded like it might make for some nice neurology. It involved a previously healthy female in her mid-twenties who had recently developed some personality changes accompanied by memory deficits and gait problems (ataxia). She was waiting to be examined back in the emergency room. Finally, Rubin got his patient to the tenth floor and took off.

Brem and Solomon had consulted by phone with Dr. Stein and with Dr. Peter Carmel, who was on his way to the hospital for the surgery. Based on what they were told, both attendings recommended a conservative approach. Though there was a piece of bullet in the center of the frontal lobes, they thought it was too risky to go after it. When Carmel arrived and looked at the patient and the pictures, he confirmed the decision. Brem and Solomon would just clean up the entry and exit wounds, removing whatever dirt, bone, and bullet fragments they could find, and then sew up the torn dura.

Remarkably, though the patient had given himself what amounted to a crude lobotomy, boring a hole right through the front of his brain, there was no intracranial bleeding that had to be stopped, and there were no major blood clots (subdural hematomas) to be removed. Since the bullet fragment was not life threatening, there was no point in attempting to remove it.

At 8:45 the first incision was made as Brem and Solomon started on the entry wound. As the operation got under way, Carmel cautioned the residents to keep things simple and to avoid taking brain unless it was absolutely necessary. "Once you start, it just keeps coming," he said and warned them that they could wind up taking the entire frontal lobes if things got out of hand.

Carmel was right at home in the OR that Friday night. He expounded on other gunshot cases he had seen, explaining the different effects produced by different-caliber guns and various types of bullets. All the while he hovered about Brem and Solomon, watching every move they made. The implication of his obsessive attention to their work was clear—even on a relatively simple case there is nothing simple about neurosurgery. "Henry," he cautioned at one point as Brem cleared the field of blood, "don't suck on that brain."

Brem and Solomon dissected the gore around the entry wound, removing one large piece of shattered bone the size of a toenail and some smaller slivers. Then, using the rongeurs, they nipped away at the edges of the hole in the skull (which would always be there). At 9:35, after sewing up the dura and closing the entry wound, they switched over to the left side of the head and went to work on the exit wound.

The exit wound was messier than the entry wound; the violence done to the brain was more apparent. Shortly

after they began their dissection, Brem and Solomon
found a jagged, pea-size piece of the bullet. It was a dull
silver color. When they reached the hole in the skull, a
little bulge of shredded brain could be seen hanging out
of the dura. "There's brain coming out," Brem said.
Carmel moved in for a closer look. The torn, bloody
tissue was an incongruous sight in a room where respect
for the smallest bit of brain was the guiding principle.
The irony of the situation was lost on no one. A man
who had tried to kill himself, who had literally blown his
brains out, was being saved.

Down in the ICU the female was dying. Carmel went
down to check on her. Surgery was out of the question,
he said, as he examined her X rays and CAT scan. "We
can't help her survive, we can only make her really bad."
In fact, she couldn't have been worse. Her brain was
virtually ripped apart by the bullet, which had traveled
up and across through the middle of her head, bounced
off the inside of her skull, and lodged in her hypothalamus, near the center of her brain. An intracranial monitor showed that the pressure inside her skull had reached
137. Normal is about 40. At that point, Carmel said, the
blood flow to her brain had probably ceased due to swelling. She was, in the words of one doctor, "organ material," a vegetable. She would die the next day, but her
organs would not be "harvested" because of her history,
which included prostitution and intravenous drug abuse.

Back in the OR, the operation on the male was coming
to an end. It was eleven-fifteen. Six hours had passed
since the patient had arrived in the emergency room, and
the system had worked for him. He had passed from chaos
to order. The prognosis was good. He would recover.
And when he awoke, everyone agreed, he would be in
for a real surprise—he wouldn't be dead.

Near midnight in the residents' lounge on the first
floor, Boris Karloff's dusty mummy shuffled once more
across a tired old TV screen, and Mitch Rubin explained
the case of the young woman with the ataxia, memory
loss and personality change. Her story was that she had
fallen out of bed a month earlier and had hit the left side

of her head, triggering five days of headaches. A CAT scan done at the time was normal. Then, in the five days prior to seeing Rubin in the emergency room, she began having memory problems and trouble walking. Her parents told Rubin that she had undergone a personality change over the last five days, particularly the last three. Basically, the changes were described as a kind of general goofiness with a lot of inappropriate laughter, alarming behavior from a twenty-seven-year-old professional. On examination Rubin found that the woman couldn't do serial sevens—counting down from one hundred by seven, that she walked like a drunk, and that she had trouble looking up during her eye exam. She was also clumsy when asked to exhibit left-hand coordination—she had trouble moving her finger from her nose to Rubin's finger and back again. (In the middle of Rubin's story, Solomon rushed through the lounge still dressed in his scrubs, including his OR booties. With a quick "Hi," he retrieved a brown-bag lunch from his room and dashed out again.)

Since the results of the tests Rubin had ordered all came back normal, he gradually eliminated several possible causes of the woman's symptoms. A new, normal CAT scan ruled out a subdural hematoma. A spinal tap and spinal-fluid analysis that proved normal eliminated viral infection. Other routine tests of her body chemistry excluded poisoning and metabolic disorders like diabetes and liver disease. Her intellect problem didn't match up with multiple sclerosis. Rubin considered the possibility that she might be faking, a psychiatric case, but, though she could have faked the memory, personality, and gait problems, it was very unlikely she could have faked her eye problem. Now, with the patient admitted, Rubin was holding out for a rare kind of viral infection that would have been missed by the regular tests; it required more sophisticated examination of the blood and the spinal fluid to be diagnosed. In addition, drug abuse was still a possibility. As he was explaining it, Rubin was clearly enjoying himself. After the gunshot wounds he was pleased to be back on some neurology. (Later, the patient admitted to periodic barbiturate abuse.)

At 1:00 A.M. Rubin was called back to the emergency room, to examine a mugging victim who had been hit on the head. The man, about thirty, was also drunk. This complicated matters, but after checking him out Rubin was satisfied that he didn't have any serious damage. Still in the emergency room, Rubin was beeped again: a medical resident wanted him to do a spinal tap on a fifty-year-old Hispanic woman Rubin had examined earlier that night. Her husband had brought her to the emergency room because she had been speaking gibberish and hadn't been able to understand anything for two days. It had seemed like a neurology case—dementia—so Rubin was called. It turned out to be a case of "raging diabetes," as Rubin put it, a diagnosis he made when he noticed that her breath smelled very fruity, a telltale sign. Her symptoms were neurological, but her illness was medical, and she was admitted to the medical ICU. Now she was to have a spinal tap, but she was still very restless, and, under those circumstances, the resident wanted a neurology resident to do the tap.

The medical ICU was older, darker, and, at 2:00 A.M., decidedly grimmer than the recently renovated Neuro ICU. The patient lay naked in her bed, her wrists secured to the bed's railing with strips of bandage. She was stuporous, half-asleep. Every now and then she moaned and moved about for a moment and then settled down again. When the doctors spoke to her, she did not respond.

The medical resident greeted Rubin with obvious relief; there was no way he wanted to do that job. But Rubin was calm and alert; tapping spines was something he knew how to do. They waited a while, for the woman seemed to be calming down. It was a long room with a row of beds down each side and a wide corridor down the middle. In the middle of the night the sleeping patients were just indistinct heads at the tops of their beds. The drapes separating them hung from the ceiling like shrouds. All around, respirators and cardiac monitors wheezed and beeped in the dark. An ICU nurse seemed to float about the ward from bed to bed, checking on her patients.

Rubin loosened the woman's right arm restraint and

turned her on her left side. The medical resident held her
hands and made soothing noises as Rubin, seated now in
a small pool of light, prepared to do the spinal tap. He
adjusted a lamp, aiming it straight at the small of the
woman's back. He was wearing surgical gloves and a
mask now, and he applied an antiseptic with a sterile
swab. All the instruments he used came from a prepack-
aged spinal-tap kit. He injected her with a local anesthetic and then kneaded the woman's back, feeling for
the right spot, counting her vertebrae until he came to
the correct interspace between two lumbar vertebrae. The
spinal cord is about one centimeter in diameter at its
largest point, encased in the hard shell of the spinal column's bones and discs. A successful spinal tap is a delicate business and not an easy mark to hit on the first
pass. Rubin took the six-inch needle and, aiming for the
spinal canal, firmly slipped it into the brown skin of the
woman's back. It was a small movement, mostly wrist,
and he did it smoothly, gracefully. It was a matter of
feel—he was looking at the spot where the needle had
entered but he was concentrating on what was happening
at the unseen end of the needle; he was in her spine.
When the needle had been placed to his satisfaction, he
drew out the wire from the middle of the hollow needle,
and a single clear bead of spinal fluid appeared. He'd hit
it on the first attempt, and his patient hadn't made a
sound. He drew off the sample they needed, removed the
needle, wiped the puncture, and put a single, flesh-
colored Band-Aid over the spot. The medical resident
said thanks, and Rubin headed back to Neuro for a few
hours' sleep.

Early the next morning, Rubin ran into some fellow
residents in the hallway as he was leaving his on-call
room. "Hey, Mitch," one said, "I hear you were scoop-
ing some brain." As another day began, Rubin stopped
and quickly told the story of his night.

III

DOCTOR

Wʜᴇɴ he was in the second grade at P.S. 18 in Queens, New York, Phil Cogen was busted by the safety patrol for drawing hopscotch boards with chalk in the schoolyard. Cogen didn't realize the other hopscotch boards for the yard were painted there by the authorities. He thought other kids had made them, and, if they could, so could he. Cogen wasn't very good at drawing the boards, and he was working on his sixth or seventh one when he was nabbed and taken to the principal's office. When he returned to his class, his teacher, whom he liked very much, told her star pupil of the possible consequences if such behavior were to continue. "Now, Philip," she explained, "it's very important that you not do this again. Because if you draw in the schoolyard, then they won't put you in the good elementary school classes, and if you don't get into the good elementary school classes, then you can't get into the special placement program in junior high. If that happens, you can't get into advanced placement classes in high school, and then you won't get into an Ivy League college and you'll never be able to go to medical school." More than twenty-five years later, Cogen still remembered how upset he was. "I thought I was screwed," he said, "I really did. But that's the way it was. I was premed in the second grade."

Cogen's ambition was instinctive and genuine. He lis-

82

tened to his teacher and spent the rest of his grammar school years living the life of the typical smart kid with no aptitude for sports—doing his homework as soon as he got home every day, passing every test with ease, and getting beat up by a lot of kids who were bigger and dumber than he was. But the physical attacks left no psychological scars, because Cogen was secure in his plan for the future, a plan that would enable him to leave his tormentors behind. And he could derive immediate comfort and a subtle revenge from the words he knew were being repeated night after night by the mothers of his classmates, words guaranteed to irritate even the most insolent young goof-off. "Why can't you be like that nice Philip Cogen? He gets hundreds on all his tests."

Cogen finished high school in three years and went on to Cornell University, where he earned an undergraduate degree in biology, also in three years. Then, when he was twenty, he did what he had been getting ready to do since the age of seven—he enrolled in medical school at New York University.

When asked why he always wanted to be a doctor, Cogen has no answer. "I don't know why," he says. "I just always did."

More than any other kind of doctor, the brain surgeon occupies a special place in the public imagination. The words alone conjure up a distinct image. He is the austere master technician whose scalpel never slips, the cold expert with the good hands. A stern mix of experience and skill, the classic brain surgeon is seen as perhaps the most professional of all professionals, someone who has seen it all. Somehow, he is even exempt from that special brand of cynicism Americans reserve for the rest of the medical profession. It is as though he were a breed apart. He may be a little less than friendly, a little aloof, but that is to be expected from a man with his responsibilities. Behavior that might be considered arrogance on the part of, say, a urologist, is likely to be excused if displayed by a brain surgeon. And this Superman of the OR has one more distinctive trait—he's old. "Always old," noted Phil Cogen, "at least in his fifties or sixties."

Phil Cogen is a brain surgeon, but he doesn't look like a brain surgeon and he knows it. Medium in height, with a high forehead and curly brown hair, Cogen is a young-looking thirty-six. In an attempt to look older, Cogen once grew a beard, but the strategy backfired. The beard softened the lines of his face and emphasized his friendly eyes, and he wound up looking even younger. Add to this his naturally cheerful demeanor and a taste for bow ties, clogs, and bright sweaters—the bow ties and sweaters being a conscious sartorial blow against the ever-lurking gloom of hospital life—and the result is a full-blown attending neurosurgeon who looks more like a resident.

In fact, for years Cogen did not consider surgery his kind of medicine. Through medical school and even into his surgical internship at Mount Sinai in New York and the beginning of his neurosurgical residency at the Neurological Institute of New York, Cogen's "concept of medicine," as he puts it, was the traditional one of the general practitioner who develops a long-term relationship with his patients and tends to all of their medical needs. During his four years of medical school he worked in the children's rehabilitation center at the NYU Medical Center, which was under the direction of the famous Dr. Howard A. Rusk. His work there, while medical, was also very social and in many respects was the antithesis of neurosurgery. Cogen, almost a compulsive talker—it never occurs to him to turn on the radio in his car and relax if he's driving somewhere with people, he'd rather talk—has considerable communication skills. His impulse is to be friendly to people, and he would probably have made a good pediatrician or any other kind of noninvasive doctor, but for one critical fact—he loves to operate.

"The thing I like best about neurosurgery is that I'm actually *doing something* to make somebody better. By taking out a tumor or clipping an aneurysm I'm doing something to improve somebody's life." It is that need to act, that surgeon's pragmatism, that eventually turned Cogen to neurosurgery. He was interested in the nervous system anyway and was considering a career as a neurologist when, in his third year of medical school, he rotated through the neurosurgery service for a week and found his calling. His feeling was confirmed when he flipped through his yearbook the next year and realized that the professors he liked the best were neurosurgeons.

After completing his residency, Cogen spent a year on the staff of Kaiser-Permanente in Redwood City, California, a private insurance hospital, before joining the neurosurgery department at Stanford University Medical Center. Cogen was on staff at Stanford for three and a half years. While there he began work on a Ph.D. in molecular biology. He then resigned from Stanford and went into the lab to prepare his doctoral thesis on the molecular biology of the meningioma, a type of brain tumor, working nights and weekends in an emergency room for income. After finishing his Ph.D., he joined the staff of the University of California at San Francisco Medical Center as a pediatric neurosurgeon.

Phil Cogen has the stop-and-go mannerisms of a man who thinks he is more relaxed than he actually is. He listens as fast as he talks, tipping his head in the direction of the speaker and freezing his ever-fluttering hands for a second as he takes in what is being said. As he gets the gist, he smiles and begins to nod. His hands resume their quick movements and you can see in his eyes that he knows what you are saying and has a ready reply. He tries not to step on the end of your sentence but he invariably does. Cogen wants to be calm and studied but he can't. He thinks too fast for that. It is not possible to take a leisurely walk with him. He is overamped; years of living without enough sleep has given him great reserves of raw energy. He is up and moving by 5:00 A.M. every day, and he often doesn't complete his duties until after ten at night, sometimes later.

All of which has helped him feel right at home in the operating suites of the major medical centers where he has pursued his career. At UCSF there are twenty ORs, where as many as fifty operations take place each weekday. All day long the halls that connect the ORs are jammed with patients on gurneys, nurses, technicians, doctors, and orderlies. The scrub sinks are crowded all the time with surgeons and scrub nurses. The procedures range from the routine to the exotic. There are liver transplants and penile implants, amputations and leg extensions. Every surgical procedure known is performed there. It's the Grand Central Terminal of surgery.

"The goal of surgery is to get as busy as you can doing good cases and making people better by operating on them," Cogen once explained. That fact used to bother Cogen, who as a resident found that, besides operating skills, the most important thing he had to learn was how to make the most of the limited time he could spend with his patients before and after surgery. "You have to learn to see people in ten minutes and make the most of it."

In many ways, the mechanics of surgery itself creates a distance between the surgeon and the patient. A patient with a tumor is a case, a collection of symptoms. He is transformed into a series of X rays, CAT scans, and angiograms—sometimes before he even meets the surgeon, who often sees the picture before he sees the patient. The patient becomes the tumor, is even referred to by his affliction. "We've got a beautiful meningioma coming in tomorrow," a doctor will say. Once in the operating room the patient disappears beneath the drapes and is reduced to a small red hole. Though it is truly the ultimate intimacy, neurosurgery can be starkly impersonal. In addition, the surgeon knows there is a high emotional price to pay for getting too close to his patients. Said Cogen, who has dreams and nightmares about his patients, "One of the things you learn to do as a surgeon in any field is to dissociate yourself from the person you're operating on. I never looked under the drapes at the patient until my third year in neurosurgery, when it was too late to back out."

During his residency Cogen took part in about seven hundred operations, and in the years since he has performed about five hundred more. In a given year, he will have anywhere from one hundred to two hundred cases. That's a lot of surgery, a lot of patients, and Cogen knows he can get only so involved. So he does the only thing possible to make up for that—he does his best in the OR.

The patient was a thirty-two-year-old woman with a pituitary tumor. Married, with one child, the woman experienced headaches, dizziness, and irregular menses.

Strangely, although she had a baby, she'd had only one period in three years. When the woman, a very religious person and a daily churchgoer, missed a day of church because of her headaches, her pastor became concerned and sent her to a doctor. Eventually she was diagnosed as having a pituitary tumor and referred to Cogen at Stanford.

Even inside the human skull, where tiny structures with outrageously complicated and critical functions are common, the pituitary gland stands out. About the size of a small grape, it is as important and, when working right, as efficient as all but a few parts of the body. As the master endocrine gland, the pituitary secretes hormones that regulate everything from fertility, growth, and skin color to the functions of all the other endocrine glands, including the thyroid and adrenal glands. Anatomically, the pituitary buds off the hypothalamus, which is one of the tiniest and most critical parts of the brain, controlling many brain and nervous system functions, including the entire autonomic system. Though not technically a part of the nervous system, the pituitary is part of the neurosurgeon's turf and can be found right at the front of the head, between the eyes and behind the nose.

To get at the pituitary the transsphenoidal approach is used. It is one of the cleanest and easiest of all the approaches in neurosurgery and it is also one of the most graphic, a kind of ultimate nightmare for people who hate the dentist. The transsphenoidal goes under the upper lip, over the upper teeth, beneath the nose, and straight back into the lower front of the brain. Save for the old transorbital approach, which was employed in lobotomy cases and involved poking an ice pick type of instrument in over the eye and through the orbital bone into the frontal lobes, the transsphenoidal is the fastest way into the skull.

For the operation, Cogen filled the OR with so much equipment there was hardly any room to move about. Besides the usual stacks of anesthesiology hardware, the large black tank of nitrogen for driving the drills, the large instrument tables, the several rolling stands that carry the power packs for the surgeon's head lights, the cautery, the three-man operating microscope, and the TV monitors—all of which were routine—two large pieces of special equipment were in the room.

Near the patient's head sat the Nicolet Biomedical Pathfinder II Evoked Potential Monitor, a rolling console with a complex-looking bunch of controls, a small green screen, and a technician. Evoked potentials are special readings of the electrical activity of the brain. Cogen was using the machine to monitor the patient's visual system during the operation. One of the serious complications of some pituitary tumors is the pressure they put on the optic nerve. In fact, it's possible for the person with such a tumor to experience an instant block of the visual pathway, to just go blind. The evoked potential monitor was connected to electrodes on the back of the patient's head, over her visual cortex, the part of the brain that processes visual stimuli. The technician also controlled a special pair of goggles the patient wore during surgery. Inside the goggles were tiny lights that the technician flashed whenever he wanted to get a reading. Before the operation began, the evoked potential reading indicated pressure on the optic nerve.

Cogen also used a Siemans Siremobile 2 Fluoroscope. The fluoroscope, which consists of a round screen monitor that looks like an ancient television set and a large armature shaped like a giant horseshoe that is positioned around the patient's head, is basically an X-ray machine that tells the surgeon exactly where in the head he is working. Because of the fluoroscope, everybody in the OR wore heavy lead aprons, some of which had plastic covers that looked like flowered curtains.

The patient lay in the middle of it all: naked, on her back, black goggles in place, looking like an exhausted pearl diver who had wandered as far from the sea as it was possible to get. As the preparations continued, she was covered with a blanket, the equipment was rolled into place around her, and the big overhead lights were brought down low over her. By the time they were ready to begin, only her nose and mouth were visible, a small circle of pale human flesh at the center of the gleaming jumble of high-tech hardware. A radio was playing clas-

sical music in the background and somebody joked about
all the equipment in the room. ''Forget the radio, let's
get a piano in here.''

The first incision was made at three-twenty in the afternoon. Cogen rolled the scope into place almost immediately and the patient's teeth glistened huge and
bloody on the color TV monitor, like something out of a
cheap horror movie. Once he had cut through the gums
and retracted everything, Cogen came upon the sella—
the small, curved bone in the middle front of the face.
The pituitary was just behind it. Using a tiny drill something like a dentist's drill, Cogen was quickly through
the sella, one of the thinnest parts of the skull. The tumor
was immediately visible, a spongy mass that, on the
monitor, looked like a tiny yellow pillow at the bottom
of a shallow bloody well. Working with chief resident
Larry Shuer, Cogen proceeded to take the tumor. Cogen
has a special interest in pituitary tumors, and he maintained a steady technical commentary as he picked away
at it.

Once in a while, Cogen activated the fluoroscope, and
a ghostly image of the patient's skull showed up in profile
on the round screen. Cogen's long, thin instruments,
poking into the head, looked black in the gray field.

After about ninety minutes it appeared that the tumor
had been taken. A piece was sent out to pathology for
analysis. The evoked potentials man reported a definite
decrease of pressure on the optic nerve. The anesthesiologist then shot eight cc's of air into the woman's head
by way of her spine. An old diagnostic technique rarely
used in the age of the CAT scan, pneumoencephalogra-
phy is often used in this particular type of case. In con-
junction with the fluoroscope, it enabled the surgeon to
get a good look at what he otherwise could not see because the opening was so small. After that, Shuer stuck
a tiny dentist's type of mirror down into the opening,
looking for any remnants of tumor.

It turned out to be a Rathke's cleft cyst, one of several
kinds of tumor that affect the pituitary. Because the tumor encased the pituitary, the gland also had to be taken.

As a result, the patient will spend the rest of her life on hormone medication.

Shuer closed up, using freeze-dried dura, fat, and pieces of bone from the opening. The dura, from a donor in Colorado, went in first, then the fat, used to pack the hole, and then the bone. As Shuer finished, at 5:20 P.M., Cogen broke sterile to call his wife, Fran, a pediatrician, on the OR phone. He was pleased with the way things had gone. "Hi," he said cheerfully. "Guess what it was?" The patient, who had told Cogen before the operation that she had made her peace with God and was ready to die, woke up fine.

Phil Cogen chose to spend his life in operating rooms and hospitals, and it is a strange life. It is strange because it is so completely different from the world outside, the rest of the world where all the people who aren't surgeons and who aren't patients spend their lives.

The tenuousness of Phil Cogen's connection with life outside the hospital was illustrated by his reaction on two occasions when he found himself out among the rest of the people in the world during the hours between dawn and 10:00 P.M. One time he took a day off during his residency in New York and went shopping on Fifth Avenue, and he caught himself looking for cases among the crowds of pedestrians. There was a woman with a suspicious-looking drooping eyelid—could have been an aneurysm. There was a man with a hint of hemiparesis; he was dragging his left foot just a bit, and his left hand was hanging oddly—could have been an old stroke. And there was a guy with the most obvious clue of all, a surgical scar clearly visible beneath a short haircut—a right parietal craniotomy. Cogen wondered what the problem had been, and who had done the surgery. Another time he found himself driving through downtown Palo Alto in the middle of the day. "It just struck me and I thought to myself, *What are all these people doing out here, shopping and driving around and everything? Why aren't they all in hospitals somewhere?*"

For Cogen, life in the hospital is what he needs and what he wants. He likes the power of being a neurosurgeon. It's there in the OR and it's even there when he asks for aspirin in a restaurant, assuring the waiter, "It's all right, I'm a physician."

One morning, there came a moment in the course of an operation that managed to capture the essence of Cogen and Cogen's job. It was not an extraordinary moment, like the clipping of an aneurysm or the opening of a spinal cord, it was a practical, unglamorous moment. But it emerged from the routine, and suddenly the key ingredient to a surgeon's success in the OR was there to be seen.

The patient had been operated on before at another hospital. He had a plastic flap in his skull that covered the old opening. The patient's pictures revealed a small tumor at the front of his brain, up against the skull, roughly between his eyes. Unfortunately, the first operation was unsuccessful; the surgeons never located the tumor. The patient, a man in his twenties, had had seizures, but his history also included an automobile accident in which he suffered a severe blow to the head. As he began the operation, Cogen was convinced that the previous surgeons had missed the tumor because they had entered the skull at the wrong spot. However, in an effort to avoid cutting away any more of the skull, Cogen at first attempted to get to the tumor using the old approach.

After cutting through the scalp, removing the plastic flap, opening the dura, and then spending an hour carefully retracting the frontal lobes, Cogen concluded that it was impossible to get to the tumor through the old opening. Stepping back, he instructed the resident working with him to extend the opening in the scalp, exposing more of the skull. Then, following Cogen's instructions, the resident took a small power saw with a handle like a black flashlight and a tiny silver blade protruding from the end of it, and he cut into the pale bone. As he guided the saw in a long arc, little clumps of bone dust collected along the edges of the new seam in the patient's skull. And that was the moment.

Strangely, the first image that came to mind was of two expert carpenters who were down to their very last piece of plywood with no hope of getting another and who nevertheless proceeded apace to cut their pattern.

The hole in the patient's head had been nearly doubled in size. The plastic flap, which he will need for the rest of his life, would now be twice as large as before, and it was Phil Cogen's decision to do it. He made it quickly, without hesitation. And in fact, it was one of the more minor decisions Cogen had made in an OR. But as the tiny blade buzzed through that skull, the simple decision suddenly seemed enormous. Cutting open skulls is part of the routine of brain surgery, but it's still extreme, irreversible, routine and radical at the same time. In this particular case, what became clear as the sawing finished and the flap of bone was lifted out was the absolute confidence Cogen had in his decision and in himself. That of course was the essence of Cogen the surgeon—his trust in himself and in his judgment. The surgeon's job is to figure out the right thing to do and then do it right. To do that requires tremendous reserves of self-confidence. The question is: Where does that confidence come from? How does it develop? How is it maintained?

Certainly, people who decide to become brain surgeons have a strong sense of self-confidence to begin with or they wouldn't even consider taking up the specialty. There are many brain surgeons, like Cogen, who don't fit the clichéd image. They are friendlier, or kinder, or funnier, or more soft-spoken than one would expect a brain surgeon to be. But there are few, if any, brain surgeons who don't believe absolutely in their skill and their ability to save lives and make sick people well again. Ego and self-confidence are job requirements. But the cockiness of a chief resident who has spent his life at the top of his class is a lot different from the self-confidence of an attending neurosurgeon who stays cool while his patient is pumping units of blood out onto the OR floor.

The first and most obvious difference is experience. "What gives me that confidence," Cogen said, "is having done this a bunch of times and having seen people do it. It's a matter of scrubbing on a lot of cases and getting a pattern in mind." That is what the residency is all about—the gradual accumulation of experience. The experience provides the surgeon with a system for approaching any given operation, what Cogen refers to as a pattern. "Each operation has its own specific series of steps," he said. "And for each kind of operation I have the steps set up to a certain point. One point being, for example, to retract the brain and expose the tumor." Along the way, Cogen explained, there are various "branch points," when decisions on how to proceed must be made. In the case just mentioned, for instance, Cogen had a plan that had to be abandoned when it became apparent that there was no way to get to the tumor by way of the original opening. His follow-up plan began with the enlargement of the hole in the skull. "You know where you're going to start, where you're going to go next, and where you're going to go after that."

A surgeon's self-confidence, then, is self-propagating. The inherent, untested confidence of the first-year resident is what gets him into the OR in the first place. Once there, he acquires the experience and knowledge he needs to operate in the methodical fashion that, if successful, increases that self-confidence.

But the key here is making the leap from resident to attending, from operating while surrounded by surgeons with years of more experience to operating alone. Beyond experience, what really separates residents from attendings is the fact that the attending ultimately has no one to turn to for help but himself. It's his show. Inevitably, something has to go wrong, really wrong, before a young surgeon can find out how well-founded his faith in himself actually is. For Cogen, the time came when he was just six weeks out of his residency.

Starting out in his own practice, Cogen said, a young surgeon is often surprised and pleased by things he tended to take for granted as a chief resident. "The first few brain tumors you do, you're amazed when you actually find it. You know, you retract and there it is and you say, 'Boy, it's really there. That's great.' " That was Cogen's experience for his first few weeks as an attending. He was working at Kaiser, operating several times a week, with plenty of variety, and he was getting good results. Because it was a private, not a teaching, hospital, there were no residents. Instead, Cogen was assisted by specially trained technicians called operating assistants.

They were good at what they did, but, as Cogen pointed
out later, "They are not people who have any actual skill
in operating that could help you." For his first three
months on staff he was being proctored by a more experienced staff neurosurgeon, who would look in on him
during the course of each operation to make sure everything was going okay.

The case that made Cogen feel "for the first time like
I really was an attending, a finished physician" was a
man in his sixties with a very large benign tumor in the
frontal lobes. "The second-biggest one I've ever done,"
Cogen recalled. "It was just a little bit smaller than a
grapefruit." The man was a quiet type of person who ran
a small business in San Francisco. His family had become concerned about him because he seemed to have
changed somehow in recent years. "He sold his store and
they retired, and when he retired his wife was real disappointed," Cogen said. "Because he was just like a
nothing. He wasn't nasty or hostile or anything. Just not
himself. So he went to see a doctor, and the doctor got
concerned because he just seemed odd. So he figured,
'I'll get a CAT scan to make sure there's nothing going
on,' and then I get this call from the radiologist to come
downstairs because the guy had a gigantic brain tumor.
Both of his frontal lobes were compressed. And the guy's
sitting there and he looks perfectly all right."

The operation was a bifrontal craniotomy. The scalp
was cut across the top of the patient's head and literally
peeled down to expose the frontal bone. That bone—his
forehead, basically—was then removed to expose the entire front of the man's brain. Cogen then retracted both
frontal lobes to expose the massive tumor. It was the
pressure on the frontal lobes caused by the mass effect
of the tumor, a meningioma, that had in turn caused the
behavioral changes in the patient. Cogen went to work
removing the tumor.

Running down the middle of the head through the dura
mater is an enclosed channel called the superior sagittal
sinus. The sagittal sinus is part of a system of sinuses
that cross the brain, serving as a drainage system. The
veins that run through the brain empty into the sinuses,

and the sinuses in turn empty into the jugular vein, which carries the deoxygenated blood back to the lungs and heart. The point is, the sagittal sinus is a very large kind of a blood vessel. The huge tumor had invaded the patient's sagittal sinus, and Cogen knew this.

"I was doing fine, this is great, no problem. The proctor was there for a while, and then just about ten minutes after he left I took out this big chunk of tumor and when I took the tumor out it pulled out of the sagittal sinus. It left a big hole in the sinus. Now, I was planning on taking the sinus, so that wasn't the problem. The problem was the guy bled two units on the floor in like five minutes."

It was a neurosurgeon's worst nightmare. Because the brain is a three-dimensional web of blood vessels, some as thick as pencils, some invisible to the human eyes, a good deal of the effort and energy expended in any brain operation is dedicated to preventing and controlling bleeding. What Cogen had on his hands was a potential disaster.

He sent out for blood and set about stopping the bleeding. "I'm piling all this gel foam on and putting on cottonoids and the thing is still bleeding and they're giving him blood. But the patient was stable, and then I got everything all packed away and I thought, *Now what am I going to do, because I'm essentially alone. I could call someone to come and help me.* But then I thought, *Let me see if I can get this straightened out myself. And if I can, then I'll do it. And if I can't, then I'll call someone to help me.*"

Cogen proceeded to ligate the sagittal sinus, stop the bleeding, and, slowly, remove the rest of the tumor. He finished at 11:00 P.M., a twelve-hour operation. Then his anxiety really began. Because the patient had been out for so long, the plan was to let him sleep through the night. That meant Cogen's normal post-op worrying time would last hours instead of minutes. The problem was, Cogen had not seen the patient's anterior cerebral arteries during the course of the surgery, and he feared that he had taken them, denying blood to the entire front of the brain. "I hadn't actually seen them," Cogen said.

"Sometimes you will and sometimes you won't. And I got real nervous that I had taken them. So I figured that this guy was screwed. But I'd done my best and I went out and talked to his family and just said, 'I think he'll be fine, we'll see.' "

During the operation, a surgeon does what he knows how to do as well as he can do it. When an emergency arises, there is no time for anxiety, no time to worry about the long-term effects. The only thing to be done is to keep the patient alive, if possible. Time stops. There is no past and no future, there is only the operation. Of course there's a price to be paid for fooling with time in such a way. And brain surgeons pay it as soon as the operation ends. Then, with the family waiting down the hall, the surgeon stands at the patient's bedside in the recovery room waiting for the fog of anesthesia to lift enough to get a response. Like Cogen, who was sure he had wiped out his patient, most brain surgeons imagine the worst as they wait for their patients to wake. In those few moments there is absolutely nothing they can do, no action they can take, and that is a state of affairs guaranteed to frustrate a brain surgeon. So they stand there, talking to their patient, watching fingers and toes, waiting for the first moan, the first rolling of the head, the first sign of life after surgery, waiting to find out if they blew it. Normally, the patient comes up enough within minutes after the surgery for the surgeon to determine the general extent of any "deficits." In this case, Cogen was forced to spend the entire night wondering how badly he had done.

When Cogen came in the next morning, the man was sitting up in bed eating breakfast. He had no neurological problems at all and left the hospital after ten days. Later, Cogen got a letter from the man's daughter thanking him for what he'd done. "We never thought we'd see our father again," she wrote, referring to his personality change. "And I remember thinking," Cogen said, *"I did it. I got this guy's tumor out and I controlled his bleeding and he made it.* That's when I started to gain confidence." A few seconds later Cogen added, "The best feeling in the world is when the patients wake up after surgery and wiggle their legs and squeeze my hand."

The pattern Cogen follows during an operation, the steps he takes and the order he takes them in, has "evolved from a series of disasters." He wasn't talking about his disasters, he was talking about everybody's disasters, a long history of disasters that has resulted in the adoption of the least disastrous techniques. Neurosurgery is a trade, learned in the operating room from people who have been doing it for a long time, and the basic rule is: Do the things that are not disastrous. Attendings teach residents to do things a certain way because they have done it and seen it done that way and they know it usually works. They may also have done it or seen it done another way, one that didn't work. The point is, not everything is written down. The lore and the literature of brain surgery spring out of the ORs, and it's all based on the simple distinction between what works and what doesn't. "The scariest thing about neurosurgery to me," said Cogen, "is that mistakes result in a screwed-up patient. I mean, if a reporter makes a mistake in an interview, as bad as it is, he can hurt somebody emotionally perhaps, or get sued. But usually nobody dies as a result of it. The same thing is true of a motion picture. You spend seven million dollars on a motion picture and it's a crappy motion picture, no one sees it, the money's lost, but no one's dead. But here, you make a mistake, you go to the wrong place, the person dies or is crippled. And that's very scary. And that's why you get into this attitude with the residents of 'You have to do it my way or else.' "

Cogen has made mistakes in the OR. "I probably have," he said. "The mistakes that I've made, though, when I've made them—and I don't think I've made too many—have fortunately been remediable to the most degree. And I always tell the patient when there's been a mistake made. People have always been very good about understanding it."

The way Cogen sees it, there are different kinds of mistakes a neurosurgeon can make. The kind of mistake he attributes to himself is "an error of judgment on something that I've thought out." It's a very different kind of mistake, he feels, from a mistake made because of negligence or ignorance. Negligence mistakes are the worst—mistakes because the surgeon was careless in some way, either in too much of a hurry or distracted or lazy or something like that, the kind of mistake that is most easily avoided. A judgment mistake Cogen explains, would be, for instance, taking too much of a tumor out, with the result that the patient winds up partially paralyzed or with some other deficit that he wouldn't have had if the surgeon hadn't tried to take so much tumor out. "In other words, you think you've got the whole thing down pat and you can see the whole thing the way it is and you act accordingly and you're wrong. But you act accordingly because you have an idea in mind." Besides this sort of error of judgment and plain negligence, there are two kinds of mistakes of ignorance, according to Cogen. "There is one which is sort of forgivable—a person who's never seen an operation done before and has prepared for it as best as possible and makes a mistake because he's just never seen it and doesn't know not to do something. And then there's the kind which are fortunately very rare—surgeons who are crummy surgeons, and they make mistakes because they just can't figure out what to do."

Because Phil Cogen is a brain surgeon he is a person nobody wants to need. The path that leads to his door is overgrown with dread. And the patient's journey, from the visit to the friendly general practitioner that doesn't follow the old routine but ends with the name and address of a neurologist, to the strangeness of the neurological exam and the frightening CAT scan, can be as terrifying as it is orderly. In fact, that orderliness itself can contribute to the patient's anxiety; dropping suddenly into the humming machinery of a medical specialty is disorienting evidence that something is very wrong. Eventually, the system brings the patient to what is perhaps the most unsettling gathering place civilized man has ever conceived—the brain surgeon's waiting room.

Time spent in any kind of doctor's waiting room is strange time. People in waiting rooms have slipped out of the healthy world and are on their way to the world of the sick. They are on the edge of that world, and there is nothing they want more than to slip right back out again, back to health. If all the minutes and all the hours that all the patients have ever spent in waiting rooms were combined, they would add up to an itchy eon of lost time, of stultifying nothingness where, if the mind functions at all, it merely drifts between idle contemplation of out-of-date magazines and morbid rumination on disease and death. Except for pregnant women looking forward to giving birth, and those chronically ill patients who have incorporated their treatment into their routine, a visit to the doctor's office is an alienating experience because it disrupts the normal pattern of daily living. Sitting in the doctor's waiting room, the patient faces the fact that his body may not be working right. Feeling at odds with one's own body is an understandable reaction to sickness, and it's one of the things that make doctors' waiting rooms such weird places. In the grip of a kind of psychological dismemberment, the patient sits there feeling betrayed by his own lungs or his own heart or, imagine it, his own brain.

Brain surgeons cut people's heads open, and nobody wants anything to do with that. And of course the brain surgeon knows it. It's a fact of his professional life that most of the people he deals with on a day-to-day basis—his patients and their families—wish they'd never heard his name. He knows that the people who need his services are probably going through the worst thing that has ever happened to them in their lives. Complicating this is the fact that what is all new and strange to the patient and his family is old and familiar to the surgeon. The patient rightly considers his brain tumor to be the most important brain tumor that ever existed, while the doctor knows that the patient's brain tumor is one of many a doctor will have to confront over the course of his career. In fact, at the outset of a case, the surgeon is probably better acquainted with the brain tumor than he is with the patient. It's an old nemesis, back again in somebody else's head. The surgeon has seen it before, and fought it before. The patient, on the other hand, is someone he's just met.

From the beginning, the patient is at a complete disadvantage. The patient is almost always new to the strange and dangerous business. While he may be frightened and shocked at what is wrong with him, the surgeon is neither; he expects people to get tumors, and he knows some of those people are going to come to him to have them taken out. Unfortunately, a bad doctor can put a patient at odds with his own body by paying more attention to the disease than to the patient.

That there is such a thing as a "surgical personality" is a fact any honest medical professional will attest to. To be accused of having such a personality is an insult to all but those who actually have them. All surgeons, by definition, do their most important work while their patients are unconscious, and it would seem unnecessary for them to have even marginally acceptable personalities. The son-of-a-bitch brain surgeon devoid of charm and bedside manner but full of OR genius, however, doesn't fill the bill, because there is more to getting operated on than just getting operated on.

Phil Cogen is nearly neurotic in his desire to be liked by the people he meets and works with. He is sensitive to the slightest of slights, snubs, and perceived insults. He obsesses about the meaning of every nod and wink that comes his way. His endless analysis of the motives and intentions of the people in his private and professional life is his least appealing trait. Sometimes it dies down a little and is barely noticeable, sometimes it's a moderate, irritating hum, and sometimes it's an exasperating rattle that just won't quit. Cogen is aware of this in himself and realizes it's not the most attractive facet of his character. Much of it is rooted, he says, in a lifelong desire "to be included. I want to be part of everything." He wants his colleagues to like him so he will feel a part of the department. He wants other doctors to like him so he'll get referrals. He wants the nurses and staff to like him so they'll do what he wants done and take care of his patients. It's all real and it's all serious and it's all a little too much. Except for the reason why he wants his patients to like him. Asked why that is so important to him, his answer is instant, short, and completely absent of any neurotic warbling. "Because they do much better that way."

So, his priorities dovetail—he wants his patients to do well and he wants to be liked and he has found that if his patients like him they will do well. And Cogen has contempt for the surgeons who allow their arrogance to infect their relations with their patients. It's one thing to engage in ego wars with other doctors, it's something else to allow your high opinion of yourself to upset your patients.

"You have to have an ego," he said. "I used to be very embarrassed about it and ashamed of it, because I was raised to be not so egotistical. But I think there's a difference between having a big ego and being egotistical. Having a big ego means that you think enough of yourself to cut into somebody's head. You think enough of yourself that you can tell someone, 'Look, I can operate on you and you'll be okay.' Being egotistical is like saying, 'I am so wonderful I am like God. I can operate on people and make them well.' It's also a matter of not being able to accept your errors. 'That couldn't have happened. I couldn't have made a mistake. Something was wrong with the patient.' "

Nobody, particularly someone who needs the services of a brain surgeon, wants to think about the fact that being a brain surgeon is a job, and neurosurgeons are like any other group, be it auto mechanics or plumbers or whatever. Some of the people in the group are very good at what they do, some are average, some are the very best, and some are the very worst. The tendency is to lump them into two large groups—geniuses and butchers.

What is easily overlooked in our impulse to either deify or condemn brain surgeons is the courage it takes to cut open somebody's head and operate on his brain. The mystery and delicacy of the brain and spinal cord are factors here—it doesn't take much of a mistake to do serious damage. "Small mistakes can kill a patient," says Cogen. "There are more little mistakes than big ones. Big ones—I mean cutting the middle cerebral artery in half or something like that—are kind of rare." Beyond the physical deficits that can result from even a successful operation—blindness, paralysis, deafness, a drooping face, a speech dysfunction—there are sometimes less tangible side effects that are completely out of the surgeon's power to control. Just about every neurosurgeon has had or has heard of a case where everything went just fine, good operation, good recovery, no apparent deficits, and then the family came back and reported that the patient was "different" after the surgery. He wasn't making a familiar gesture anymore, for instance, or his laugh just wasn't the same—strange, elusive changes in behavior that only close friends or relatives could ever pick up on. No apparent cause, save that the person had his skull opened and his brain handled.

The point is, the brain is very much an unknown quantity, and it takes a lot of nerve to cut on it. It takes courage. Even so, perhaps it isn't such a serious thing, the way the courage of neurosurgeons is overlooked, or taken for granted. For one thing, the money and prestige that go with the job are substantial. For another, anything that keeps a neurosurgeon's ego in check is probably for the best. And finally, as every surgeon knows, the bravest person in any operating room isn't the one with the scalpel in his hand; it's the one on the table.

IV

PATIENT

THE frightening thing about many of the disorders that require brain surgery is the way they strike—suddenly and at random. It could happen to anyone at any time. Brain tumors and seizures come out of nowhere and change everything forever. They trigger a flow of events that may later seem organized and even orderly but which constitute in fact one long emergency. Those afflicted find themselves plunged into chaos and adventure.

This is the story of Gail Kraley, whose brain malfunctioned. She isn't typical, she doesn't represent anything, except for the simple truth that every human nervous system is a person and every person is an individual. The details of her case are unique, as she is unique. On the other hand, she went through something that thousands of others have gone through, so she is one of many.

All brain surgery patients wind up with a story to tell, and though each story is different, most of them have one crucial factor in common—they begin at some specific point in time and space. The patients know exactly when and where it all began, the very moment when they first realized that something was going on and they didn't know what it was.

Young, pretty, and nervous, Gail was on the first big assignment of her new job and she didn't want to blow it. At the age of twenty-two she had already made the huge professional leap across the Hudson River, going from a daily newspaper in her home state of New Jersey to a Manhattan-based magazine covering the advertising industry. She was bright, talented, and ambitious, and she also had that special savvy that people get when they grow up in the shadow and under the spell of New York City.

She was to write an in-depth feature article about a woman executive, and she was starting the preliminary interview, trying to look alert and ask insightful questions, when she noticed that her left hand was falling asleep. She was writing on a legal-size yellow pad with her right hand, and without looking down she began to wiggle the fingers of her left hand, which she believed was lying in her lap, underneath the pad. Nothing had ever fallen asleep on her quite that way before; it was just dead weight, and the sensation upset her. Somehow, though she knew what kind of pad she was using, she decided she was using a spiral notebook and that she had gotten her fingers caught in its wiry spine. As she continued to look straight ahead and concentrate on the interview, she tried to work her fingers free, but it was no good and the feeling persisted. Finally, she looked down at her lap. Her left hand was not underneath the pad as she had thought; it was lying there, well away from the pad, curled up into a claw and the fingers were twitching. As she watched it, it curled up even more, bending at the wrist, the fingers twitching uncontrollably. It was the weirdest thing she had ever seen, and she felt a surge of adrenaline as she stared at her own hand, fascinated.

Gail grabbed her left hand with her right hand to try to stop the twitching as she told the woman executive that something strange was happening.

"What is it?" the woman asked, coming around the desk to sit beside her and look at the hand.

"I don't know," Gail said, "this has never happened to me before." As she continued to clutch her hand, Gail, mortified and convinced that the woman whom she had just met thought she was some kind of freak, apologized for the scene she was making.

After about forty-five seconds the twitching subsided,

though the numbness, which had spread up her forearm, remained. Just then, her left upper lip started tingling and went numb, as though she had been given a shot of Novocain. The numbness spread up under her nose, down to her lower left lip, and then to her gums and the left side of her tongue. Focused on her mouth, she forgot about her hand for a moment. Then she thought of her hand again, and it was as though it had nothing at all to do with her; from the middle of her forearm down it was divorced from the rest of her body.

Gail immediately thought she had cerebral palsy, multiple sclerosis, a stroke, or a brain tumor. It looked like palsy, and years before she had known someone with MS, though she had no idea what the symptoms were. A brain tumor also seemed an obvious possibility. And when the numbness spread to her mouth, she thought of a stroke. She thought she was about to lose the entire left side of her body. But even as these fears ran through her mind, she couldn't really believe there was anything seriously wrong at all.

Just minutes after the onset, the woman executive's boss came into the office to say hello. Hiding her left hand behind her back, her mouth still numb, Gail shook hands with the man and tried to keep the small talk to a minimum, afraid that if she tried to smile or say too much the left side of her mouth wouldn't operate. Then the woman told Gail there was a meeting they ought to attend. "If it's okay with you," Gail said, "first I'd just like to call my doctor and let her know that something really bizarre just happened."

Actually, Gail's reference, "my doctor," wasn't accurate. The doctor was in fact her father's doctor, and Gail had been to see her only once before, three days earlier. Feeling even flakier than she had during that visit, Gail called the doctor and explained what had happened. The doctor told her to come in right away. Gail resisted. She was feeling okay, though her hand was very tired, and she was reluctant to leave her assignment even for a little while. It had taken her a long time to set it up and it was off to a bad enough start already. When Gail insisted, the doctor agreed and told her to come in as soon as possible, sometime in the next couple of days. Gail hung up and went back to the interview. Twenty minutes later the numbness started again.

This time she paid closer attention to it. It started in her thumb, then spread to her other fingers and went up her arm. This time the fingers didn't curl up but felt as if they were electrical, as though they had some kind of a charge running through them. Again, her mouth went a short time after her hand and arm. Though she had remained calm the first time it happened, calling on reserves of professionalism to maintain her composure in front of a stranger, she became panicked this time. She was fairly hysterical when she called her father at his Manhattan office; he told her to slow down and tell him exactly what was happening. "I don't want to slow down and tell you what's happening," she said. "I'd like you to get here, and I want to go to the doctor. I'm not going to take time out to explain what's happening while my hand is going berserk."

By the time she and her father got to the doctor's office, her hand and her mouth had improved. The doctor examined her and found everything to be normal but told her that the problem was definitely something neurological. Gail's main concern was that nothing permanent happen to her hand. "It's not in your hand," the doctor said, "it's in your head." The doctor told her to see a neurologist as soon as possible and instructed her to call immediately if the symptoms recurred again. Then, determined to do her job, Gail had her father drive her back to the advertising agency, where it had all started. She apologized profusely and finished the day without any more problems.

That night, instead of going back to the apartment she and her sister shared in Manhattan, she went to her parents' home in New Jersey, just across the George Washington Bridge. She, her two sisters, her brother, and her father were sitting around in front of the TV set discussing what had happened when it started to happen again.

Gail called the others over. It started in her thumb and spread to the other fingers and then went up her wrist. The numbness quickly began to feel as though there were something shooting back and forth inside the hand, beneath the skin. The fingers didn't curl up, and though they felt to Gail as if they were twitching wildly, nobody could see anything happening. Her family looked and put their fingers on the hand, but they couldn't feel anything. Then Gail didn't want them to look at it anymore—she thought it too repulsive, even though the hand looked normal. A few moments later, as it had the other two times, the numbness went to her mouth.

Gail didn't want to call the doctor right away; she wanted to have dinner first. After all, it wasn't really anything serious. But then, five minutes after the onset, the numbness and buzzing went straight up her fingers, through her arm, and on up to her shoulder. When it got to her shoulder, she thought it wasn't going to stop until it got to her heart. She thought she was going to have a heart attack. Finally, it stopped at her collarbone. She was badly frightened but not crying.

That was a Monday night. A CAT scan and an EEG were scheduled for Thursday. Gail worked Tuesday and Wednesday, and things were fine. Thursday she took the day off and, accompanied by her sister Lauren, went to the Columbia Presbyterian Annex in midtown Manhattan for the tests, still believing it was nothing serious, just a fluke thing they could all laugh about later.

The EEG is a peaceful sort of a medical procedure. It was the first one they did that day. Electrodes were attached to various spots on Gail's head, and she was instructed to lie very quietly in the dark for a while and to doze off if possible. With the machine humming and nothing happening, Gail found it very pleasant in an odd sort of way. Except for the gluey conductor paste in her hair it wasn't bad at all. After a while the technician got her up in a chair and had her hyperventilate. Gail didn't like this part of the exam. The woman giving the test was too cheerful, in that phony way so typical of medical technicians, and she wouldn't tell Gail anything about the readings she was getting. After hyperventilating for a while Gail was told to stop, and the woman asked her how she felt. "I feel fine," she said. And within seconds her thumb started to go.

The twitching quickly spread halfway up her arm, and Gail, for the first time, started to cry. She cried because it seemed the technician had somehow caused the new incident. As the technician rearranged the electrodes, placing one on the thumb, trying to get everything recorded and all the time asking Gail not to cry, Gail's nose, lips, and tongue all went numb.

Then the technician left the room to call a neurologist, and Gail, who was still crying, became even more upset. *Don't leave me here,* she thought, *with this seismograph going and my head hooked up and my fingers twitching and my lips numb.* She knew they knew something she didn't know.

Her sister came in, and Gail calmed down after a couple of minutes, and then the technician returned to disconnect her from the machine. "What is it?" asked Gail.

"Well, I'm not the one who can tell you that," the woman answered.

"Well, obviously you're looking for something, right?" Gail said.

"Yes," the woman said, "the doctors are looking for something but I can't be the one to tell you." That aggravated Gail and insulted her, and she felt a sudden urge to punch the woman and make her talk.

She was sure that she had a brain tumor. She washed the conducting paste out of her hair in the sink—things were bad, but she wasn't going to walk around with glue in her hair—and by the time she had ridden the elevator from the fourth floor to the basement, they were all ready for her at the CAT scanner, and that made her even more nervous. Several people came out to greet her, all cool and professional.

"So," Gail said, "you guys know what you're looking for, right?"

"Oh yes," said the woman in charge, "we have some ideas. Now take off your earrings and lie down on the table and we'll talk about it later." *Oh great,* Gail thought, *I'll lie down on the table, you'll send me through this giant tunnel thing, you'll zap my brain cells with whatever is coming out of that machine, and you know what's going on and I don't.*

The CAT scan went smoothly, except for one moment when Gail coughed a little and everyone came running out of the control room to see if she was all right. Their attention made her wonder just how sick she was. It took about forty minutes and when it was over the woman came out with the pictures and told Gail that she had already talked to the neurologist.

"Oh," said Gail, "so you found something?"

"Yes," the woman said.

"Is it a brain tumor?" Gail asked.

"No," the woman said, "it's an AVM." Gail had never heard of an AVM, but she didn't have a brain tumor, and that was something.

Gail was taken to another room, where she got on the phone with the neurologist her doctor had referred her to. It was strange; Gail had never met the person and now she was talking to this stranger about a thing in her head called an AVM. "I can't promise that's what it's going to be," the neurologist said, "but that's what it sounds like to me." The neurologist explained what it was, and Gail asked if it was going to kill her or cripple her. By the time she was off the phone she knew she wasn't dying and she also knew that she might have to have brain surgery. She had an appointment to see the neurologist at eight the next morning.

After they left the Annex, Gail and Lauren stopped at a store in their neighborhood and bought thirty dollars' worth of fancy candy and ice cream and then went home to their apartment to watch television. They had Gail's CAT scans, and they held them up in front of the television to look at them. And there it was, a strange blob in the middle of her head that was actually blood, the remnants of a cerebral hemorrhage. Gail thought it looked huge.

The next morning, Gail, her sister, and her parents went to the Neurological Institute of New York to meet the neurologist. She was no-nonsense and gave Gail and her family straight answers. As she examined Gail and took her history, Gail remembered something. From the start of the seizures, her father's doctor and the people at the Annex had been asking her if she'd had any head trauma in the past, any kind of incident that she could recall, and she had told them all that she couldn't think of anything. As the doctor asked the question again, Gail remembered that when she was about twelve, at summer camp, she had come down with a terrible headache that had turned her into a "crying mess." She was given Tylenol with codeine, and she had spent the day resting. When the neurologist heard this she nodded and said, "That was it, that was the first hemorrhage." Then she said that they couldn't be sure if the blood showing on the CAT scan was from the old hemorrhage or the new hemorrhage.

The preliminary decision was that surgery would be advisable. After Gail argued for one more week of work in order to get her story done, she was scheduled for admission on the Friday of the following week. To control any future seizures, she was put on Dilantin, a powerful anti-seizure medication. Gail took ten pills the first night, in a standard dosage plan known as top-loading. At home in Manhattan that night, after taking seven pills, Gail was gone, bombed, and she was worried about taking three more. She called the hospital and was told by a resident on duty to follow her doctor's orders, so she took the other three, and when she woke up the next morning she was as wiped out as she had ever been in her life. She could barely lift her head off the pillow, she was dizzy, her limbs were twitching. She got hysterical and called the hospital again. A neurology resident told her that she had in effect been poisoned and that it would take forty-eight hours for the medicine to be out of her system.

Two days later Gail went back to work. During a lunch interview she felt her thumb start to go, and she panicked. "Excuse me, I gotta run," she said, horrified at the thought of another seizure right there in the restaurant. She had learned a little more about the seizures, enough to fear that they might get larger, and she pictured herself flopping around on the floor.

In spite of what she now knew about her condition and that she was probably going to have brain surgery, Gail was still not thinking of her problem as something that

was wrong with her brain. Though she had begun to
worry about grand mal seizures, she was primarily tar-
geting her hand. Even in her worry about the seizures,
she managed to keep her mind off her brain; her chief
concern was the indignity of it, the embarrassment. She
couldn't tolerate the thought of being unconscious and
having her body jerking about while other people
watched.

She got through the week with no further problems—
the twitching of her thumb in the restaurant didn't progress in the usual pattern—but her story about the woman
executive was not coming together. She was past her
deadline and worrying about it when she went into the
hospital.

A friend of hers had had knee surgery and had spent
some time in the hospital. He told Gail, who had never
been in a hospital before, to prepare to lose her dignity.
"Just leave your dignity at the door and you'll be fine,"
he said. She couldn't accept that.

Her hospital roommate was a twenty-seven-year-old
epileptic, and Gail could not relate to her at all. The
woman seemed out of it, Gail thought, and she blamed
it on the fact that the woman had been taking a variety
of anti-seizure drugs for years. As she learned more about
the woman's medical history, and as she watched her
submitting to the tests and swallowing the pills without
saying a word, Gail decided the woman was a basket case
who deserved what she got. Above the woman's bed,
taped to the wall, were tongue depressors and an airway
gadget in case the woman had a seizure. The sight of
them revolted Gail, and she couldn't stand the fact that
she had to share a room with the woman. They had nothing in common, she thought, and then she remembered
that they were in the same hospital. She softened a little,
but the whole setup still gave her the creeps.

Gail was scheduled for an angiogram the next morning, and she was petrified, primarily because she knew
she would have to be awake for it. The night before, a
woman had come to shave her pubic hair and though Gail
had thought it would be traumatic, it wasn't. She merely
wondered what kind of job it must be to go around shav-

ing people's pubic hair off. Then a resident came in to take her history and do a neurological exam. Gail thought he was brusque and she didn't like him very much. All the time he was with her he kept getting calls about another patient, who was having a bad time of it, and Gail was struck by how cold he was about it. He left for a while, complaining about having to go to resuscitate an old lady yet again. When he came back he gave Gail the "doom and the gloom," as the residents call it, explaining to her about the nature of her disorder and the possibility of stroke, paralysis, and death. When he left, Gail blamed herself—she had asked the questions, he had just answered them.

The next morning, after watching *I Love Lucy*, Gail climbed up on a gurney for the ride to the basement. She didn't like the idea of the stretcher and insisted that they set it so she could sit up on it, rather than ride lying down. She'd put on one of the infamous hospital gowns with no back, and as she bumped through the halls it occurred to her how odd it all was, to be riding around on that thing with her pubic hair shaved off, a patient at the Neurological Institute, someone who needed brain surgery.

The basement was busy as usual; the hallway was jammed with people in wheelchairs and on stretchers, with babies, in rolling cribs. Gail noticed that the babies were having a fine time, but the adults all seemed nervous.

A major diagnostic tool in the treatment of cerebrovascular disorders, an angiogram involves the injection of radioactive dye into the blood supply of the brain. A catheter is run into the femoral artery in the thigh and then threaded up through that blood vessel. When the injected dye enters the brain, an X ray is made showing the brain's blood vessels in great detail.

Gail was heavily sedated, but she didn't feel she was sedated enough. There were four or five people in the small room with her, and an X-ray machine above her head. The first step was a shot of Novocain in the area of the artery—a needle in the groin, basically—and that wasn't as bad as she had imagined it was going to be.

Then, with Gail straining to see what was going on, they ran the catheter. A resident was doing the work, and he was being talked through it by an attending. Throughout the procedure the staff kept asking her how she was, using terms of endearment like *honey* and *dear*. At one point, she saw a squirt of her blood as they cut into the artery with a scalpel. Then she felt a strange pressure as they ran the catheter into the artery; for some reason it reminded her of fishing tackle, as though that was what they were running into her groin. In spite of the sedation and the Novocain it hurt, a persistent discomfort aggravated by the fact that it was all going on in her groin and she just wanted it out and over with.

They ran tape across her forehead and chin to hold her head in place. Then they all left the room. When they shot the dye it felt hot above her eye and above her ear. They had to shoot it twice to get it right. When they had finished, they took her across the hall into a supply room and removed the catheter. Then someone sat for twenty minutes pressing on her artery to stop the bleeding. Then they stuck her out in the hall again and warned her not to move around or the bleeding would start again. She was spaced out, lying there in the hall, when her neurologist came by and said hello. Then they came and took her back to her room.

She was dopey and sore and didn't want to use a bedpan. She was incapacitated for the first time in her life and she hated it. She had visitors and she wanted to be up and about and entertaining, but she had to lie there like a sick person.

That night Gail and her family were told that she was being discharged. The angiogram revealed that it might not be possible to remove the AVM. There would have to be some discussion, and the surgeon her neurologist wanted to consult was out of town. The news didn't bother Gail as much as it bothered her parents. Gail just wanted to get out of bed and back to real life. But her father was upset at the possibility that the thing was inoperable. Gail didn't think about that. The neurologist talked with Gail about the likelihood that she might start to feel depressed because she was in a situation where she was forced to confront her own mortality. And Gail said, "Who's facing their own mortality? I'm not facing any mortality."

And the doctor said, "Well, I'm telling you not to worry if that's what happens. It's very common." Which did in fact disturb Gail, but she fought it, thinking to herself, *Well, you think about my mortality. I'm not thinking about it. There's nothing wrong with me, honey.*

She went home the next day, a Sunday, nearly two weeks after the first seizure, expecting to go back to the hospital on Saturday. Then, on Friday, she found out that the surgeon consulted had determined that the AVM was operable, but the surgery would not take place for ten days. Gail finally got upset. She did not want to spend another ten days walking around, waiting for another hemorrhage, worrying about having a big seizure while she was at work. Everything was in disorder; her story still wasn't finished, and the Dilantin had caused a rash all over her body. Things had been going so well lately; the last thing she had expected to defect on her was her brain. But it had. Now all she wanted was to get on with the surgery and get it behind her.

One week later she had a second CAT scan, this one at a special angle as requested by her neurosurgeon. An hour after that she and her parents finally met her neurosurgeon, Jost Michelsen. Michelsen, an ex-Marine and an ex-Harvard quarterback, has a rich, commanding voice. He is a recidivistic cigarette smoker, and when Gail met him he was smoking again and she liked that, because she was a smoker too. She wanted to like him and she did. She wasn't too worried; she had gotten used to the idea of brain surgery, and she also figured that at least half of the doctor-patient relationship was in her control. By the time she got to Michelsen's office Gail had already gone and had her hair cut short. She had done that herself because she wanted to feel that she was running things. She felt the same way that morning—taking "her" CAT scans, going to see "her" neurosurgeon and asking all the questions. It was her brain, her operation, and as far as she was concerned, her show.

Michelsen explained to Gail that she had a capillary

angioma, a tight, almost tumorlike ball of tiny blood vessels. He told her that it was easier to take out than an AVM and more dangerous to leave in, and he gave her an article he had written about cerebrovascular surgery. Gail asked how soon after the surgery she would be walking, and he said the next day. He said there might be a residual problem with her left hand, but that if there was one it would probably clear up without special therapy. He told her the angioma went an inch deep into her brain and said the question about whether it could be removed was raised by the fact that they weren't sure if the thing was being fed by a major artery. That was not the case, in his opinion, although there was no test to prove it, because the angiogram didn't work on capillary angiomas. That was why he had ordered the second CAT scan, to get a better look at things. He also mentioned that there was a chance there would be a tumor, but, again, he didn't think so. Gail asked what the risks of the surgery were. He said the one that really had to be considered was the risk that she would hemorrhage on the table and die.

It was an honest, frightening answer, and Gail quickly decided she would worry about it later. Though Michelsen had raised the specter of her death, it wasn't real to her. So she liked him, with his hardy style and his can-do attitude. The meeting was more like a chat than a conference, and he answered her questions and her parents' questions to their satisfaction. Before she left his office, it crossed her mind to toss him a pen to see if he caught it or to have him write his name to see how steady his hands were, but she didn't do those things.

The following Wednesday, almost a month since the first incident, Gail went back into the hospital. Her operation was scheduled for the next morning. Her new roommate was a spinal patient with a pack of Marlboros by her bed, and Gail was relieved to see that. She got right on the phone and called all her friends and gave them her number. Then a resident came, a different one, and Gail had him do a full neurological exam so her mother could see what that was like. Then a medical student came in and told her she was going to observe the operation and how excited she was about it, because it was such a "weird condition." She used the word *weird* several times, and Gail said, "Don't tell me how weird it is. I don't want to know that it's weird. I want to know that it's common." Gail asked the student to watch everything and report back to her. She wished that she could see it herself, she said. Actually, she said, she didn't want to see, she wanted to oversee. It bothered her that she would never really know exactly what went on in the operating room. She had a lot of company the night before the surgery, and she got a lot of toys, including a ray gun that she used to zap whomever and whatever she didn't like.

When visiting hours ended, she insisted on being taken up to the ICU, where she would be going immediately after her surgery. A young woman who had had brain surgery that day was sleeping, but the nurses told Gail that she had just been up talking with her parents. They offered to wake her up again to talk to Gail if she liked. Gail got a kick out of the ICU nurses. They gave her a tour of the unit, and she felt healthy and normal. Then she saw the babies in the pediatric ICU and she felt foolish for being nervous. There was an infant sleeping there and Gail thought, *Well, if this kid can go through it, so can I.* Altogether, the ICU wasn't so bad; gross, Gail thought, but not horrible. "That's fine," she said to the nurses, "I've seen it. There's nothing more I can do up here now but lie down in a bed."

Gail went to sleep that night with no problem and, looking back, she could not believe it. "I must not have been thinking," she said later.

Gail had asked her sister Lauren to be there when she woke up the next morning, and she was. The rest of the family arrived about 7:45. Her nurse had had an aneurysm operation, and that morning she had Gail feel the holes in her head. Gail was given Valium and a shot, and Gail was gone. Then the transport people came, and Gail moved from the bed to the gurney, embarrassed about the flap in the back of her gown. She waved good-bye as they wheeled her out of the room.

From the start, one of Gail's major concerns was her

hair. As soon as she heard the words *brain surgery*, she was thinking *bald*. Her family and her friends told her she was silly to worry about it, but she worried nonetheless. So, her hairdresser was in on it from the start. Gail had her hair cut to what everybody thought the shaved part would look like three weeks after surgery. And she told Dr. Michelsen that she wanted as little as possible taken off for the surgery. She worried about her hair so much because she couldn't believe that anything else would be wrong with her when it was all over.

The orderly who cuts the patients' hair is a friendly man who does his best to make the patients happy. He followed Gail's instructions and shaved as little as possible on the right side of her head as she lay on her gurney in a tenth-floor prep room. Then Michelsen came by and patted Gail on the hand and said, "I'm sorry, but we're going to have to take a little more." When they wheeled her into OR, Gail wanted to sit up and take a good look around, but the anesthesiologist was ready and she went under so fast she didn't even remember where they stuck her.

The operation went well, and it was over in less than four hours.

Gail's family came to see her in the ICU, but she was still pretty well out of it. Only their faces registered with her. Michelsen came by a little while later, and she was more awake. "You're all right," he said, "it went well."

"Is it what you thought it was?" she asked.

"Yes," he said.

Besides her hair, one of Gail's other big worries was her appearance immediately after the surgery. She had told Lauren that under no circumstances was she allowed to let her look disgusting if she was not capable of taking care of herself. "I am not going to look like one of those shriveled-up lumps," she said. "Position my body. If I'm not doing it already when you get there, put on my makeup and mascara. I do not want to look sick and debilitated." When her sister came back at seven-thirty that evening, Gail, who was feeling fine, noticed that she kept stepping out on a small terrace off the ICU. Lauren told Gail later that the sight of the drains coming out of her bandage—two thin plastic tubes that carried a light flow of blood away from the wound in her scalp—made her so nauseated she couldn't stand it.

Later that night they brought in another patient and put her in the bed opposite Gail. The nurse told Gail that the woman was very sick and there was a chance she wouldn't make it through the night. "Now look," Gail said, "if she's not going to make it through the night, I want you to promise me that at some point you're going to come over and tell me that she's dead or dying. Because I don't want to be lying here without being able to see what's going on and have this woman die right across from me. I do not want that woman to die without someone coming and telling me, 'Hey, she's dead.' "

Gail slept through the night with no problem. In the morning a nurse came and pulled out the drains, which hurt a lot, but Gail was so surprised to learn she even had them hanging out of her head that she didn't yell much. Then they pulled her IV and her catheter and sent her back to her room in a wheelchair.

She put on a T-shirt and a sweatsuit and checked herself out in the mirror. With her turban in place, she thought she looked pretty good. *Look at me,* she thought, *brain surgery doesn't look too bad.* She had a new roommate, with serious back pain, who was moaning quite a bit. Gail felt okay. That morning she took some Tylenol and that was it.

The day after surgery she had a dozen visitors. Her roommate was in pain and crying, so Gail took her guests down the hall to the solarium. Throughout that weekend Gail carried on like a hyperactive child. She had droves of visitors. She couldn't stand to be alone, she couldn't sit still and watch television, she couldn't rest in her bed and read. She played with her toys and roamed up and down the hall visiting the other patients. Everybody knew who she was, the funny girl with the sunglasses and the Donald Duck hat that squeaked and the laser ray gun for zapping people. No one would ever had guessed she'd just had brain surgery.

Monday morning Dr. Michelsen showed up and said, "Let's take those bandages off." Gail panicked for a minute. She was all by herself and she didn't want to be alone when the bandages came off. But they were off in seconds, and she didn't even have time to get to the telephone.

Because she was doing so well, her parents and her sister had gone back to work. Her mother was coming for lunch, and because Gail knew the bandages were coming off that day she had asked her to bring a scarf. But Gail hadn't expected Michelsen so early. Now, there he was, looking down at her and beaming. ''Hmmm, looks good,'' he said, ''looks good.'' She was afraid someone would come to visit her before she got the scarf.

She went to look in the mirror, and it was what she expected; she was expecting something disgusting, and she thought it was disgusting. She had twenty-seven staples in her head. Her scar was pink, new, and curved like a small horseshoe back in an arc from the mid-front of her head down to a point just above her right ear. She sat on the edge of her bed and watched people pass in the hall. She was afraid that the other patients would be upset with her because she was sure she had convinced them that there was nothing wrong with her. She looked in the mirror again and thought it was gross but not devastating. Then her mother came and she handled it just fine—her mother didn't act upset at all. Gail put on her scarf, and visitors came, and she entertained all day as usual. But she felt odd, naked.

That day she got yet another new roommate—the woman from the ICU who hadn't been expected to make it. The woman was in bad shape, strapped to her bed, mumbling and rambling, and she thought it was 1949. Gail did not want to deal with her. She wanted to get out of there. She did not belong. the others were sick and she was healthy. In a way, Gail felt it was cruel of her to be so healthy. On the other hand, all she could do was flaunt it. They had opened her head and operated on her brain, and there she was in her sneakers running around the hall. She took a shower by herself the morning after the operation. She cut herself shaving; that was her big problem.

She had talked to patients and their families about what

miracles they were performing at the hospital, like some kind of goodwill ambassador. She had followed the nurses around, talking to them, and relating to them because she refused to think of herself as a patient. *I do not want to be associated with the sick and the terminally ill and the wretched and the moaning,* she thought. But now there she was, with that scar. That night, Monday, she started crying, and she couldn't stop.

She woke up Tuesday morning and sat up in bed and started crying. She cried all the way to the shower, in the shower, and all the way back. She cried because she was bald and because there was nothing she could do about the fact that she was bald. She cried because she had an incision with twenty-seven staples on her head. She cried because they had performed brain surgery on her and because everybody was thanking God she was healthy and didn't die or have a stroke. She cried because she was luckier than her roommates and the other patients around her and she didn't feel lucky. Until the bandages had come off she had done a good job of convincing herself and everyone else that having brain surgery was like going to the manicurist—no pain, no fuss, no muss. And then she was bald, with a scar, and she was repulsed.

Gail was released from the hospital five days after the operation. Her family gave her a homecoming party, complete with presents for the patient, and Gail had a fine time. Then, over the next few days, with everyone gone back to work and school, Gail was alone more often, and her mood turned black. She had never felt so awful in her life; she almost didn't feel human. Her family, thrilled at how well things had gone, tried to cheer her up, but she wouldn't cooperate. She couldn't understand how people could sit down at the dinner table and eat with her. One of her first days at home, before she could wash her hair, she was eating lunch, alone in her parents' house, and for an instant the idea occurred to her that she didn't have the right to eat; how dare she be doing something so normal, she who looked so abnormal. She cried for a week.

The irony was that in the annals of neurosurgery, Gail

was a booming success. Everything went as planned, and she woke up with no deficits. The potentially deadly capillary angioma had been successfully removed. She was a nice, clean case with good results and a great prognosis. And she couldn't stand the sight of herself.

Gradually, over the course of the next two weeks, Gail came to terms with the sight in the mirror. Her hair was growing back much slower than she had expected, but she finally accepted the fact that there was nothing she could do about that. Then she realized she would be going back to work soon, and she had to deal with everybody seeing her, with her scar and her peach fuzz patch. So she did what came naturally, she made a party out of it, inviting her friends from the office to her apartment for cocktails so they could get a good look at her and get used to it. Then she started going out in public without her scarf. She went to the bank and the supermarket and the dry cleaners, and she got a lot of stares, but she felt better without a scarf or hat hiding things. She was nervous as hell, smoking a lot of cigarettes and talking constantly, but she wasn't crying.

She didn't think about the fact that the surgery had saved her life because she never really felt that her life was in danger. Her hand had been twitching, and her mouth had been numb, but she never really made a connection with her brain, with the inside of her head. Her ability to speak and to think weren't affected, so it was easier for her to see it as a hand problem. When she thought of her brain she thought of cognition, logic, reason, and those things had remained intact.

In the weeks after the surgery, Gail was eager for her next appointment with Dr. Michelsen, to find out what had gone on during the operation. She wanted to know everything that had happened, and she wanted to know if she had looked dignified on the table. She also wanted to know if she was going to have more seizures. They had told her that there was nothing else wrong with her brain, that there were no tumors or aneurysms or any other surprises, and so she felt pretty assured that her brain wasn't going to blow again. But she wanted to hear it all one more time.

Three weeks after surgery the patch over her scar was still downy and new and the scar was clearly visible, though it wasn't raw-looking. It was thin and pink. Her hair strategy had been a failure, and that bothered her. And then she got an idea. Even if she couldn't make the stuff grow any faster, it was, after all, her head; she was in charge of it and could do whatever she wanted with it. So she did. She dyed it. But not all of it. She dyed just a small clump, right on the crown of her head, a bright orange. It stood out like a tiny flag in the middle of her shorn brown mop. And now there were two things to notice about the pretty young girl with the short hair.

Part Two

BEYOND THE KNIFE

V

DISORDER

As harrowing as her experience was, Gail Kraley was lucky in one sense—her problem was not a mystery, and her treatment was clear-cut and direct. In fact, she was a "good case" because she was young and healthy and her preoperative workup left little doubt about what the surgeons would find. The risks, though substantial, were the routine risks of brain surgery. Unfortunately, to appreciate the ironic luck of neurosurgery patients we have to compare them to others who are not so oddly lucky, and in the world of neurological medicine such people are not hard to come by. Only a small minority of neurological cases lend themselves to surgical intervention. The majority are beyond the reach of the neurosurgeon, in the complicated, often mysterious, and sometimes strange realm of the neurologist.

Amyotrophic lateral sclerosis (ALS), aphasia, and schizophrenia are three disorders that affect movement, language, and thought, three nervous system functions so basic they are inevitably taken for granted. These are not rare disorders. ALS, the least common, afflicts thirty thousand people in the United States at any given time; aphasia is a problem shared by an estimated 1,000,000 Americans; schizophrenia strikes fully one percent of the world population.

Each disorder provides insights into the practice of neurological medicine and the nature of three essential

125

nervous system functions. Our knowledge of the underlying anatomy and physiology, the types of treatment involved, and the relative level of sophistication of the affected nervous system functions are different in each case. Though much is known about the parts of the nervous system involved in movement, including the part of the system ALS destroys, the actual cause of the disease is unknown. There is no cure, and the treatments are limited to symptoms only. The language function is the best understood of the higher cortical functions; and aphasia, which usually results from stroke, is often treatable with rehabilitative speech therapy. Schizophrenia, on the other hand, involves the nervous system's least understood parts. Although today's treatment is certainly better than it was forty years ago, the drug therapy involved is relatively crude, given the sophisticated nature of thought, the highest of the higher cortical functions.

In combination, ALS, aphasia, and schizophrenia offer a vivid portrait of the noninvasive side of neurological medicine. They define its limits and they embody its potential. The patients, families, doctors, nurses, and researchers involved with the disorders live in a world where the rules can change, where nothing can be taken for granted, where walking, speaking, and thinking are not the sturdy elements of everyday life they seem to be, but fragile and extraordinary gifts that can be lost.

VI

MOVEMENT

IMAGINE that you cannot move. The next time you have an itch, stop a moment and imagine that you cannot move a muscle. As the itch spreads, imagine that you cannot turn your head or tap your foot or even speak aloud. Remain immobile, concentrate on it, and if the itching gets bad enough maybe your eyes will tear, and if a tear runs down your check you won't be able to wipe it away. Imagine that you cannot even swallow your own saliva. You are completely paralyzed; you are not being restrained, you are not tensed up, there is simply no energy there. You can feel things—the itches, the cramps, the full bladder—all the usual sensations are coming through loud and clear, but the motor pathways to your muscles have shut down, and you are trapped in a kind of physical silence, a profound and complete stillness of body. Now imagine that the thing that has taken away your ability to move is also killing you, and it is doing so with dispatch; after a couple of years of total paralysis you will be dead.

All movement depends on a kind of nerve cell called a motor neuron. Motor neurons are well described by their name. Their job is to carry the motor impulses from the brain through the spinal cord and out through the peripheral nervous system to the muscles. They are critical links in the chain between the mind and the body.

Motor neurons are the opposite of sensory neurons, which receive and conduct sensory information to the brain.

Amyotrophic lateral sclerosis, better known as ALS and best known as Lou Gehrig's disease, is a neuromuscular disorder in which the motor neurons degenerate. As a result, the muscles atrophy and the patient becomes paralyzed. It is a progressive, terminal disease that usually strikes people in their fifties and sixties. More men than women get it, by a ratio of about two or one. About 4,600 new cases are diagnosed in the United States each year. The earliest symptoms of ALS are almost perversely minor—weakness in a finger, a twitching muscle in the forearm—an onset so insidious that the first signs are often overlooked or mistaken for some other problem. (The fact that the disease usually strikes older people, who often have other complaints, exacerbates the problem of early diagnosis.) As the disease progresses, the muscles, no longer innervated by the motor neurons, waste away. Usually, only the muscles of the eyes are spared. Eventually, patients are unable to swallow or even breathe on their own. Death is often the result of respiratory failure due to muscle weaknesses. The disease is painless, and the brain itself is unaffected. As the body dies, the intellect remains intact. Average life expectancy is about two or three years.

ALS was first identified in 1869 by the French neurologist Jean-Martin Charcot. Though the disease's cause and cure are still unknown, current researchers are exploring a handful of theories, ranging from a virus, to an autoimmune system failure, to some kind of heavy metals poisoning. Currently, no theory carries more weight than any other, and the field is wide open. ALS is a classic example of "selective vulnerability," because it affects only motor neurons. The mechanism of the disease must therefore be extraordinarily specific and subtle, at least as subtle as the biochemical differences in the various types of neurons. An analogy would be a type of rust that could bring down a bridge by destroying only the rivets that hold it together, while leaving the beams and cables intact.

Three different forms of ALS have been identified.

Guam-type ALS is found on the West Pacific island of Guam, where the incidence of the disease among the native population is one hundred times what it is for the general population. Hereditary ALS, which accounts for 5 to 10 percent of all cases, is a form of ALS passed from generation to generation of the same family. Sporadic ALS appears randomly in the general population. In addition, it is generally recognized that ALS has three different rates of progression: the typical rate, in which the patient survives two to three years; an accelerated rate, in which death occurs within a matter of months or even weeks; and a very slow rate, in which the patient survives for ten years, twenty years, or even longer.

The fact that ALS is known as Lou Gehrig's disease is a terrible irony. Far more than most people, Gehrig based his life on his ability to move, and to move well. The thing he did best, hitting a baseball thrown by a professional pitcher, is considered the single most difficult feat in sports. It combines concentration, coordination, balance, timing, and strength in a classic American burst of energy. It amounts to a showcase for all the amazing and routinely overlooked elements of movement. In one sense, Gehrig's was the very first case of ALS; certainly, it was the first case of Lou Gehrig's disease. The details of that case, the details of Gehrig's life and death, reveal the essence of ALS—devastating and total in its power to destroy, cruel and relentless in the way it destroys.

Lou Gehrig lived the kind of life millions of American men have dreamed about, a life of spectacular accomplishment on the baseball field. It was an exciting life, filled with home runs and World Series games and shared with such fellow New York Yankee legends as Babe Ruth, Miller Huggins, Joe McCarthy, Bill Dickey, and Joe DiMaggio. It was a rare life, a long dream of summer that stretched on, hit after hit, game after game, season after season. Gehrig's greatest record, the feat that defined him as a man and as a ballplayer, was a matter of endurance and consistency—he played in 2,130 consecutive major league games over a span of fifteen seasons. To the fans of the day it must have seemed that Gehrig would play forever, that his phenomenal strength and skills would always keep his name in the sports pages. Surely he was the man who would one day possess a whole string of records as the oldest this and the oldest that— the oldest player to win the batting title, the oldest to be named MVP. But it didn't work out that way.

The life that so many envied, that great life playing ball under the sun, had a proportional strain of tragedy quietly hissing at its core. Gehrig's motor neurons degenerated, and he was gone. The end was as fast and mysterious as the career had been long and simple (simple in the way the game is simple, the way a curve ball is simple, if you ignore the physics). When he lay dying at the age of thirty-seven, just two years after his illness was diagnosed, the Iron Horse was weaker and more helpless than an infant, unable even to swallow a mouthful of water. He left a double legacy, as a baseball hero and as the victim of a strange and terrible disease. The greatest first baseman of all time wound up as a landmark case in the annals of neurology.

Though he died a comparatively young man, just shy of his thirty-eighth birthday, Gehrig has, for several reasons, always seemed older. For one thing, he was a ballplayer, and thirty-seven *is* old for an athlete. Also, from the vantage point of the late 1980s, newsreel footage of Gehrig and his teammates has an ancient look to it. The flickering shades of gray age everyone. The styles of the day are also a factor. In his baggy wool uniforms Gehrig looks like a hulking middle-aged man instead of a strong athlete. And the consecutive-game streak also contribute to the sense we have of him as an ancient—anyone who played in all those games must have been old.

But Gehrig was not old, and to understand and appreciate what happened to him, we have to keep that in mind. We have to picture him as he actually was—young and in color, one of the fittest members of his generation, out there every day playing baseball on green grass, under blue skies. We have to think of his incredible streak of games not as an insurmountable statistical mountain, a monolithic *thing*, but as many smaller things, as individual games, each complete unto itself. We have to think of them as 2,130 separate events—2,130 opportunities for Lou Gehrig to enjoy himself and play his game. And what a game it was.

The thing about the streak is that it wasn't *the streak* for many years. Gehrig played the early part of his career free of the renown that went with the streak. What made him famous in the beginning was his incredible talent for producing runs. Long before he dominated the sport as the Iron Horse, he dominated it as Larrupin' Lou, cleanup man in the Yankee lineup known as Murderers' Row.

Gehrig's stats are so far above today's standards that they boggle the mind. Gehrig wound up with a career batting average of .340, which tells us that when it came to seeing the ball and getting his bat on it, he was one of the best of all time. But it was the kind of hits Gehrig got that made his name—the long kind, the kind that scored runs.

Scoring runs is the diamond-hard fact at the center of baseball, and Lou Gehrig was a run-producing machine. He drove in more than 100 runs thirteen years in a row. In seven of those years he topped 150, including 1931, when he drove in 184 (the American League record and second best—to Hack Wilson's 1930 mark of 190—of all time). Not counting his three partial league seasons (1923, 1924, and 1939, which totaled only thirty-one games), Gehrig averaged 141 runs batted in (RBI) and 134 runs scored for fourteen years. And he did this batting right behind Babe Ruth for ten years, and Ruth's own amazing ability to drive in runs undoubtedly cut into Gehrig's totals.

What Gehrig's numbers finally define is an overwhelming offensive force, a masterful presence in the batter's box, a slugger who consistently generated action on the field. When he swung his bat, he blew the elegant geometry of the game to pieces; he hit 493 home runs, which the carefully placed defenders could only watch, and 535 doubles and 162 triples, which sent those defenders charging into the empty places on the field, where

Gehrig's rockets bounced and rolled to the wall. When you think of Gehrig, you should think of a field with all the players running as hard as they can—some on the way to score, the rest in a rush to control the ball.

Gehrig's career was one of great seasons, great games, great moments. On June 3, 1932, he hit four home runs in a nine-inning game, a feat only two other players had accomplished (Robert Lowe in 1894 and Ed Delahanty in 1896). He was the MVP twice, in 1927 and 1936. In 1927, besides driving in 175 runs, Gehrig hit 47 home runs and had a batting average of .373 and a slugging average of .765. That was the year Ruth hit his 60 home runs, and what has often been forgotten is that for most of that season Ruth and Gehrig were neck and neck in pursuit of the home run title (they were tied as late as September 5 with 44). In 1936 Gehrig hit 49 homers, batted .354, and drove in 152 runs. In 1934 he won the Triple Crown.

In spite of what he did with his bat, Gehrig became best known for the consecutive-game streak. And that's probably the way it should be, because the streak was as much a result of his personality as it was of his endurance and skill. He was a hardworking man whose low-key style stood in sharp contrast to Ruth's. Playing first base for the Yankees was his job, and it was there that he established himself as the Iron Horse. He played with broken fingers, pulled muscles, and crippling back pain. He played in spite of beanings and who knows how many other routine aches pains. He played with Ruth and, a decade later, he played with DiMaggio.

When a baseball player is in his stance at the plate, awaiting the pitch, his entire nervous system is on full alert. His cerebral cortex, the largest part of the brain, is originating motor output and processing sensory input, and the hitter may even be using it to think. His cerebellum, a large, semidetached part of the brain located at the back of the head, is involved in the maintenance of equilibrium, muscle tone, and posture control. The batter is receiving sensory information from his visual system, from his inner ear, and from sensory nerves known as proprioceptors, deep in his muscles and joints. These are the nerves that provide the hitter with his sense of body awareness and movement. The player's spinal cord is flashing with nerve impulses to and from his brain.

When the pitch is thrown, his nervous system goes into high gear as he makes his split-second decision to swing. He follows the ball with his eyes as it comes toward him and begins to bring the bat around; and as he does, he makes adjustments in his body, arms, and legs even as he continues swinging. Sensory information is still coming in and being processed as he carries out an explosive voluntary motor function. If everything goes right, he hits the ball.

A superb athlete like Gehrig, acutely attuned to the condition of his body, must surely have picked up on the earliest signs of ALS. And just as surely, he must have dismissed them as something minor, something that would just go away.

The disease killed Gehrig's game before it killed Gehrig. As early as spring training in 1938, more than a year before the end of the streak, observers noted that Gehrig didn't seem to have the old power anymore, and his numbers for his last full season support that. He finished 1938 with a batting average of .295, 29 home runs, 115 runs scored, and 114 RBIs. Today, such a season would qualify a man as a million-dollar player, but for Gehrig it marked a serious drop in production.

As the 1939 season began, sportswriters knew that the end of the streak was near, and they knew it was going to be a big story. They watched Gehrig closely, and what they saw from spring training on was far worse than anything they'd seen the season before. He couldn't hit the ball and he couldn't play defense. "Yankee followers were amazed to see how badly Gehrig had fallen from the peak," *the New York Times* reported later. "He was anchored firmly near first base and only the fielding wizardry of Joe Gordon to his right saved Gehrig from looking very bad." Offensively, Gehrig had trouble getting the ball out of the infield; his line drives had become pathetic pop-ups.

Gehrig opened the season at first base, and the streak continued for eight more games. But they were sad affairs. In the first game of the year, against the Boston Red Sox, the opposing pitcher, Lefty Grove, walked DiMaggio in order to pitch to the punchless Gehrig. It was an incredible thing to witness; no pitcher had *ever* wanted to see Gehrig come to the plate. It was the ultimate insult, sure proof that the Gehrig of legend was no more. To make matters worse, the strategy worked. Gehrig hit into a double play.

Over the course of those final eight games Gehrig got just four hits—all singles—and one RBI, while batting .143. The end came after a game against the Washington Senators on April 30. Four times Gehrig came to bat with men on base, and each time he failed to get a hit. He stranded a total of five base runners as the Yankees lost by a score of 3–2. For Gehrig the RBI man, that, combined with an overenthusiastic response by his teammates to a routine play in the Senators game, was enough. The next scheduled game was in Detroit on May 2, and for the first time in fourteen years the Yankees took the field without Lou Gehrig in the lineup.

The end of Gehrig's consecutive-game streak was national news for days as sportswriters around the country analyzed his career and his sudden fall from the top. The consensus was that Gehrig had simply worn himself out. DiMaggio's opinion was that Gehrig had squeezed as many as nineteen years of work into his fourteen full seasons in the big leagues. A *Boston Sunday Globe* story quoted a ''leading Boston osteopath'' who theorized that ''Gehrig's case might be due to some toxic condition started by a case of grippe in the winter.'' In the same article a psychologist said that a hitting slump such as the one Gehrig was experiencing when he ended the streak fit the description of ''an occupational neurosis.'' The article continued, ''When this came on top of worry about his record, self-examination as to whether he was earning his high salary, and doubt whether he should continue the daily grind, it is easy to see how Lou— even-tempered as he is—might have been thrown temporarily into a nervous and mental tangle.'' Another theory was that Gehrig had "caught" something during an all-star tour of Japan in the fall of 1934. A doctor who had been treating Gehrig routinely for some time was convinced that it was a gallbladder problem, while Gehrig's wife secretly feared that her husband had a brain tumor.

Gehrig himself attributed his problems to the cool weather of the early season and to the lumbago that had been bothering him off and on for years. He was looking forward to the warmer months, fully expecting to get back into the game. "My immediate plan is to try to regain my old form," he said a week into his new life in the dugout. "Sitting on the bench I have a lot of strange thoughts and peculiar sensations. But I do not sit there with the idea that it is all over and Gehrig is ready for the boneyard. Not by a long shot."

Gehrig never played in another regular-season game. His last appearance as a baseball player was a three-inning stint in an exhibition game with the Kansas City Blues, a Yankee farm team, in early June. From Kansas City, Gehrig went to Rochester, Minnesota, and checked into the Mayo Clinic. He knew something was wrong, and he wanted to know exactly what it was.

In the library of the Baseball Hall of Fame are Gehrig's scrapbooks, two huge volumes containing newspaper clippings, postcards, snapshots, letters, and telegrams. The black fabric covers are embossed with LOU GEHRIG in faded gold. The scrapbooks are arranged chronologically, and deep in the second volume is the single sheet of paper that transforms the hero of the previous pages into the victim of the final pages. It is the press release issued on June 19, 1939, Gehrig's thirty-sixth birthday, by the Mayo Clinic. A masterpiece of understatement, its five sentences officially ended Gehrig's career and foretold the end of his life. It reads, in its entirety:

TO WHOM IT MAY CONCERN:

This is to certify that Mr. Lou Gehrig has been under examination at the Mayo Clinic from June 13 to June 19, 1939, inclusive.

After a careful and complete examination, it was found that he is suffering from amyotrophic lateral sclerosis. This type of illness involves the motor pathways and cells of the central nervous system and in lay terms is known as a form of chronic poliomyelitis (infantile paralysis).

The nature of this trouble makes it such that Mr. Gehrig will be unable to continue his active participation as a baseball player, inasmuch as it is advisable that he conserve his muscular energy. He could, however, continue in some executive capacity.

Signed
Harold C. Habein, M.D.

The news that Gehrig was suffering from some strange disease revived and amplified the shock that accompanied the end of his playing streak. At the same time it explained the mystery of his collapse as a ballplayer, and as so often happens when a diagnosis is made, it brought to light previously overlooked symptoms. Eleanor Gehrig recalled that she had noticed Lou stepping off the curb in a strange way that spring, his foot sort of plopping down, as though he were blind and not sure about the curb's height. She also remembered some uncharacteristic falls he took while ice skating the previous winter. His teammates remembered stumbles and even a fall Gehrig took while leaning over to tie his shoes in the clubhouse. And the sportswriters finally put their fingers on the elusive nature of Gehrig's problems on the field earlier in that year—he'd lost the "spring" in his muscles.

Though he was seriously ill, Gehrig nevertheless was relieved to know that something beyond his control had taken away his game. The deathwatch that spring, with the reporters following him around and asking him how he felt all the time, waiting for the inevitable end of the streak, had been hard on Gehrig. The reporters had been waiting for Gehrig to drop into the ranks of the mortal, of the typical thirty-five-year-old athlete who just doesn't have it anymore. But Gehrig had been too good for too long, and he was too proud to accept that. He had to have known that there was something extraordinary about his sudden fade, and when the disease was diagnosed his idea of himself as someone special remained intact.

When he left the Mayo Clinic, Gehrig rejoined the Yankees and remained with the team for the rest of the season, performing the ceremonial task of taking the line-up card out to home plate before the start of each game. It was a poignant time, filled with standing ovations and feature articles in the local papers. Many of the articles focused on a whole new angle, Gehrig on the bench and the man was amiable and enthusiastic on the subject.

"So help me, for fifteen years I never saw a ball game as it should be watched," Gehrig said in June, soon after his diagnosis. "I never appreciated some of the fellows I've been playing with for years. What I always thought were routine plays when I was in the lineup are really thrilling when you see 'em from off the field."

Gehrig's approach to the disease was equally optimis-tic. From the start he told everyone that the doctors had given him "a fifty-fifty chance to fight this off in two years," though it seems unlikely that the Mayo Clinic doctors would have told an ALS patient any such thing. In her memoirs Eleanor Gehrig wrote that, on her in-structions, the doctors did not tell Lou the whole story. She was told that the disease was fatal and that her hus-band had about two and a half years to live, but she said Gehrig was told only a very basic version of the infor-mation contained in the press release and was apparently allowed to develop the idea that the progress of the dis-ease could possibly be arrested.

However, according to one former Mayo staff member, Gehrig did know the fatal prognosis. But he carried on. He maintained a regular correspondence with the physi-cian who diagnosed him and was interested in the state of research into the causes of ALS. He also made contact with others suffering from the disease and even under-went a series of experimental treatments—injections of vitamin E directly into the muscles. But as the 1939 sea-son wore on, Gehrig developed a limp, and the weakness in his hands became more pronounced.

Diseases of the central nervous system were certainly something new to the sports beat and, not surprisingly, mistakes were made. The most common one was confusing ALS with polio, and the Mayo Clinic statement was partly to blame for that. There was also a lot of corny writing—ALS was described as "the toughest pitcher [Gehrig] had ever faced," and more than one writer noted that if the first baseman could beat the disease he would "score his greatest victory." At the same time, there were some simple yet astute descriptions of Gehrig's problem. "The muscles were there, but there was no nerve energy behind them," wrote one reporter, which is both clear and accurate. On August 8, 1940, the New York *Daily News* ran an article that sought to account for a Yankee slump by raising the possibility that Gehrig had infected the entire team with polio. Under the headline HAS "POLIO" HIT THE YANKEES? and a lurid illustration showing a player in a Yankee uniform collapsing in a landscape reminiscent of a World War I battlefield under gas attack, ran such prose as "They played ball with the afflicted Gehrig, dressed and undressed in the locker room with him, traveled, played cards and ate with him. Isn't it possible some of them also became infected?" Gehrig sued the paper for one million dollars, an enormous amount at the time. Almost as soon as the piece came out, the Yankees began a surge that carried them from fifth place into the pennant race, and when the paper published an apology, acknowledging that there was no evidence that ALS was communicable, Gehrig dropped the suit.

After the 1939 season Gehrig accepted a job as a member of the New York City parole board. He officially assumed his duties in January 1940. Gehrig took the job seriously, reporting for work each morning at his office in the municipal building and making regular trips to the city prisons to interview inmates. A frequently published photograph from that time shows Gehrig seated at a paper-strewn desk in a suit and tie, looking like a sharp and healthy young executive. But the photograph was a lie; to a trained eye, the telltale atrophy of the muscles in his hands and face is apparent. Within months of starting the job, Gehrig's arms were so weak he couldn't lift his hands off the desk. As his condition worsened, he gave up the job and went into seclusion at home, where he saw just a few select friends.

Gehrig died at home on June 2, 1941, sixteen years to the day after he began his consecutive-game streak. A few years after his death his wife appeared before the U.S. Senate subcommittee to plead for funds for research. In her testimony she summed up what had happened to her husband. "At first," she said, "he simply couldn't play baseball with the skill which won him a place in the Hall of Fame. Then he couldn't play well enough to stay in the Yankee lineup. Finally, he couldn't play baseball at all. As the disease progressed, he couldn't dress himself, he couldn't feed himself, he couldn't walk."

The obituaries and editorials on Gehrig flooded the nation's media, and for the next two years he was honored in various ways, most often by having something named after him. Signs bearing the words LOU GEHRIG FIELD went up on previously nameless baseball diamonds in towns and on military bases around the country. In addition, the Yankees retired his number (the first time that it was done in baseball) and erected a monument to him in center field.

The disease took his name as well. Amyotrophic lateral sclerosis stripped Gehrig of his magnificent skill as a baseball player, killed him, and got itself a new name in the process. And because the term Lou Gehrig's disease is so common now, it's easy to overlook just how odd that is. Most diseases either have technical names, like poliomyelitis; have names related to the symptoms, like scarlet fever; or are named for the man or men who first identified them, like Alzheimer's and Parkinson's. Gehrig is the only individual patient to have a disease named after him. Although it began as a reflection of Gehrig's fame, the name shift also testifies to the eerie power of ALS to consume its victims. When it consumed Gehrig, it also consumed his career. As a result, one of the greatest baseball players who ever lived is best known for the way he died.

Lou Gehrig didn't just get ALS, he *became* ALS. And while his case is exceptional, it's a good example of the multifaceted nature of serious disease. A disease is many things. It is a group of related symptoms as well as an underlying organic disorder that causes the symptoms. A disease is a foreign thing, and also a natural process arising in the patient's body, a part of that body. ALS was the death of Gehrig, and it was a terrible death. But it was also part of his life, and that was a positive life even as it came to an end. In the face of this disease Gehrig displayed dignity and optimism, a dignity and optimism perhaps best exemplified by the eloquent speech he made at Yankee Stadium on Lou Gehrig Day, July 4, 1939, when he said he considered himself "the luckiest man on the face of the earth."

Another kind of eloquence best ends the story of Lou Gehrig. It is found in a headline that ran on the back page of the New York *Daily News* the day after Gehrig was honored at Yankee Stadium. It reads: YANKS SPLIT, LOU WEEPS WHILE 61,808 FANS CHEER. That does it. It captures the ironic tragedy of it all with just the right mix of baseball and reality, business as usual and business not so usual at all, with a stat, of course, to hold it all together. The Yanks win one and the Yanks lose one, and Lou is gone and the game goes on.

The great thing about baseball is the way it never ends; there is always another inning, another game, another season. And Gehrig, better than anyone else, understood the beauty of that idea, and the power of it. Nothing strange, nothing mysterious, just keep playing and try to win more than you lose. The only real mystery of Lou Gehrig's life was the mystery of his death. Everything else was as clear and as simple as a line drive on a sunny day.

Interestingly, fear and ignorance of ALS persisted in baseball for years. "Doc Cramer keeps telling me that if I go on catching every game I could get the sickness that killed Lou Gehrig," Yankee catcher Yogi Berra said in the summer of 1953. Berra was discussing the endurance of players of different generations with teammates and a reporter. When the reporter said to Berra that Gehrig died "not by overwork but by a paralyzing bug," Yankee shortstop Phil Rizzuto responded with a theory that others in the sport had propounded at various times. "But how do you know that Gehrig's incredible record didn't have something to do with his death? I believe that by playing every day through nearly fifteen seasons, whether he was well or ill, he invited trouble. He must have weakened his resistance and left himself wide open for the disease which strangled him."

Of course, baseball players and reporters were not the only ones who had wrong ideas about ALS in those days. Doctors, too, came up with some bad theories. In 1943, a Philadelphia surgeon, believing that pressure generated by varicose veins within the spinal column caused the degeneration of the nerve cells, developed what he considered a potentially effective operation for the treatment of ALS. The surgical treatment involved cutting away parts of some vertebrae in order to decompress the spinal cord. After performing the operation on three patients, the doctor reported improvement in two of them. No evidence to date supports the theory.

Because there is still no cure, the ultimate fate of an ALS patient is the same now as it was in Gehrig's time. Indeed, until recently, the day-to-day details of the typical patient's life after diagnosis were also the same as they were fifty years ago—unrelievedly grim. ALS patients were considered hopeless cases and were sent home to die. In spite of the Gehrig connection, ALS remained an obscure disease in the public mind; his death may even have contributed to that. The only thing people knew for sure about ALS was that it had killed Gehrig and done it in a strange way. It was perceived as a rare disorder, and it did not attract the kind of research funding made available for more widespread diseases. With no relief from the medical establishment and no understanding among the public, ALS patients endured their suffering alone. In desperation, some resorted to quackery; snake venom injections were the most popular of the bogus treatments. They didn't work, of course, but they offered ALS patients something precious and rare—an option.

Today, thanks to an increasingly organized ALS community made up of patients, their families, and the health care professionals who deal with the disease on a regular basis, there are a number of new choices that ALS patients can make. While ALS remains a terminal disease with a tragically short life expectancy, there is a growing feeling among those involved with the disease that the care and treatment of ALS patients should focus on the quality of life, not the length. Lynn Klein, director of patient services for the ALS Association, a national health organization that raises funds for research and maintains a network of patient and family support groups, is well aware of the medical establishment's traditional view of ALS as a death penalty. "So many times patients will tell us that when they were diagnosed, the doctor said, 'You have ALS. Go home and get your affairs in order, you're going to die in two to five years.' We are working very hard to change that attitude."

Having worked as a nurse for twenty years, Klein understands how ALS can bring out the worst in a doctor. "Remember," she says, "physicians are trained and schooled to heal. You give a pill, you perform an operation, you give radiation treatment, you give chemotherapy. You do something for that patient and make him well. With ALS, the doctor is faced with his own mortality, his own inability to cure, so he pushes it away."

Klein spent thirteen years working in hospitals as an obstetrics nurse before going into home care. When she met her first ALS patient, it changed her life. He was a thirty-four-year-old man with two children the same age as her own. "One month into the case, I knew I never wanted to do any other kind of nursing," she recalls. "I saw the devastation of the disease, and it became such a challenge to me. Here was a disease for which there was no treatment, no cure; they didn't even know what caused it, and yet here was this man fighting. He couldn't move a muscle and he was fighting for his life. It gave me such a good feeling that I was able to contribute and help him. I just got ALSed."

Because most ALS patients remain at home, at least until the final stages of the disease, families are intensely involved in the care of the patients, and it can destroy normal home life. Klein thinks of family members as "the unrecognized victims" of ALS. "It just takes over the whole house," Klein explains. "A patient can become totally paralyzed and dependent on life-support systems and live that way for many, many years. The wife of one of my patients, after a year and a half, was coming unglued. And they had a fairly good marriage. She said to me, 'Lynn, he's either got to get well or die. I can't keep going on. This is like limbo.' They had no sex life, they had no social life. Her life consisted of going to work, coming home, and being there for her husband."

Klein's assessment of the impact of ALS on families is borne out at the family support group meetings the ALS Association helps to organize. They are searing, emotional sessions where the husbands, wives, sons, daughters, brothers, sisters, and friends of ALS patients share their feelings and experiences. At one such meeting, held in a community hospital in California's San Fernando Valley, a woman in her thirties described the effect of her father's illness. Her mother had been sleeping on the floor next to her father's bed for three and a half years, and the mother's anger and frustration had all been turned against the daughter. "Our relationship is nonexistent," the daughter said. "To my mother, I'm the enemy." Another woman told how her mother's ALS was affecting her seven-year-old son. "I just don't have time to do all the things we used to do together," she said. "I can't be the mother to him that he needs me to be." To care for her mother, the woman and her son had moved out of their own home and into the grandmother's home, and the boy had been forced to change schools. To make matters worse, the grandmother was in full denial and refusing to take meals with the rest of the family because she was embarrassed about the problems she was having with her swallowing. Still another woman, a nurse in her early twenties, tearfully described how her family had drifted apart when her father contracted ALS and her brothers and sisters had let the weight of his care fall to her. A gentler note was sounded by a woman whose husband was afraid that people would think he was drunk when he began to have trouble walking as a result of ALS. "He took my arm, and that's the way we have walked ever since," she said.

The idea behind the modern "management" of ALS—Lynn Klein's preferred term—is to treat the symptoms of the disease as aggressively as possible, whatever they may be. That means exercise and special diets to maintain strength, drugs to control routine medical problems like excess saliva and muscle cramps, speech therapy and computers to facilitate communication, and psychological counseling to deal with the emotional problems faced by the patients and their families alike. The emphasis is on living with ALS, as opposed to dying from ALS. Former United States Senator Jacob K. Javits, of New York, was diagnosed with ALS in 1980. Javits spent the final years of his life drawing attention to the disease and to the plight of the terminally ill in our society. He engaged in an active search for the meaning of his life and of the lives of others, sick and well alike. Addressing a group of doctors in 1984, he summed up his hard-won philosophy. "If there is anything I can leave you with in terms of the treatment of patients with terminal illness, it is this," said Javits, who spoke from a wheelchair while a portable ventilator aided his breathing. "We are all terminal—we all die sometime—so why should a terminal illness be different from terminal life? There is no difference."

Lance Meagher is the embodiment of Javits's words and of the new attitudes taking hold in the ALS community. He lives on a wooded hill on the coast of Oregon, in sight of the Pacific Ocean. It is a place where nature displays a large and powerful aspect. Great forests run right down to the churning, rocky coastline where cold white waves leap and roar. When the night is clear, a shining universe of stars hangs thick in the sky; some few, hanging low, nearly touch the sea, while others, in clusters, blur together in streaks. When the fog comes, it drops quickly and rolls onto the shore, hugging the ground and smothering the lights in town. It is a resonant setting for Meagher, who is a different kind of product of nature.

Meagher was diagnosed with ALS in 1977 at the Massachusetts General Hospital. He was thirty years old. It was a confirmation of a diagnosis the young doctor had made himself a year earlier, an instant diagnosis he arrived at on rounds one morning in May 1976 when a muscle in his arm began to twitch. "I looked down at my biceps," he recalled years later, "and I immediately thought, *ALS*." He knew it was ALS, though it could have been any number of things, including a simple, benign muscle twitch, and he knew what it meant—that he would be dead in three years.

For nearly a year Meagher kept his knowledge to himself and went about the business of completing his residency in internal medicine. (Neurology was a specialty he didn't like at all.) He kept himself too busy to think about what was happening to his motor neurons, spending long hours on call in the hospital, moonlighting a second job, and playing the violin in a classical music group to fill whatever spare time he had left. But then the disease began to progress, and when it started it was his violin playing that was the first thing to go. Next, his handwriting began to deteriorate, and when people began to notice that something was wrong he went through the steps of confirming what he already knew.

Less than two years after the official diagnosis, the disease began to pick up speed. At the beginning of 1978 Meagher was fit enough to go skiing, but by the end of that year he was in a wheelchair. He stopped practicing medicine, but his life went on, and he got married in the fall of 1980, by which time he was quadriplegic. Seven months after he got married he reached the point where he could no longer breathe on his own or swallow well enough to eat or drink. In April 1981 he was hospitalized for a tracheotomy and a pharyngostomy and became completely dependent on life-support systems. A ventilator breathed for him, and he received all of his food in liquefied form through a tube that entered the side of his neck and ran down through his pharynx and his esophagus and into his stomach.

Meagher thought he was going to die soon, and he and his wife made all the preparations. They also decided to have a baby. Although it never worked out, Meagher believes that the decision to try is the reason he is still alive thirteen years after contracting ALS—a longevity that qualifies him as a medical marvel and a de facto ALS expert. In the course of events that followed, he discovered that he had a low sperm count. Although he received nothing but discouragement from the fertility experts he and his wife consulted, Meagher pursued the problem and eventually established that his low sperm count had a fairly rare cause—a very low count of a hormone called follicle stimulating hormone, better known as FSH. In December 1982 he began injecting himself with FSH three times a week as a treatment for his infertility. In just a short time he noticed that his prime ALS symptom—muscle fasciculations (twitching)—decreased. He continued with FSH, increasing the frequency of injections to every other day, and the progress of the disease slowed and then ceased.

While Meagher believes the FSH arrested the progress of the disease, others disagree, and there are cases of ALS where the disease seems to simply burn itself out, which could account for Meagher's results. To test his theory, Meagher stopped taking FSH for five months, from November 1986 to April 1987. He found that his symptoms and deficits increased while he was off the drug. When he resumed the injections, he found that the symptoms decreased again in two weeks.

As a doctor, Meagher understands the need for proper studies, and as an ALS patient he also understands the need to avoid raising false hopes. Most of his evidence for FSH is anecdotal. Inspired by his own success with the treatment, Meagher resumed his medical practice in 1987. (The FDA approved FSH as an experimental treatment in ALS in April of that year.) Meagher sees only ALS patients. After a year back in practice he reported that of two dozen ALS patients he had seen who were using FSH, "about half believe their disease has significantly slowed or almost stopped its progression, and the other half believe there has been no progression."

Meagher does not know how many ALS patients around the country are using FSH, which costs about thirty dollars per shot, but he gets calls from doctors and patients all the time who have heard about the drug and are eager to try it. He is eager for a large study to be done, complete with all the usual controls and protocols, and has been lobbying a number of research institutions to undertake the project.

When he is working on research, Meagher thinks of ALS in terms of pathophysiology; he thinks about degenerating motor neurons and his belief that the disease is linked somehow to a dysfunction of the pituitary gland, a dysfunction that might in turn be caused by an infection of some kind, a very specific infection that destroys certain pituitary cells. "But most of the time ALS is just a very large, nebulous cloud which you are always in," he says. "Even so, it does not have to affect your day-to-day living." In addition to his FSH work, Meagher has evolved an overall approach to life with ALS. Based on his own experience, it forms the basis for his renewed medical practice. His new patients come and stay with him for a two-day seminar, during which he introduces them to his ideas. Meagher emphasizes general good health based on good nutrition and a realistic acceptance of the limits imposed by the disease. "Without doubt, most people who succumb to ALS die of infection and not just from ALS," he has written in one of his papers. "Healthy, well-nourished people are much better equipped to fight any type of infection. It is sad that most people with ALS have such a heroic attitude that they want to eat by the customary oral route, no matter how much time or discomfort is involved. I have yet to see anyone who has the least trouble eating maintain a sufficient caloric intake, though they often believe the contrary. Although a natural response, denial will adversely affect one's health, and should be watched for."

Meagher knows that a lot of ALS patients resist feeding tubes and even ventilators until the last possible moment because they believe that by accepting them they are surrendering to the disease. "But it's really just the opposite," Meagher says. The way he looks at it, an aggressive approach to dealing with ALS means accepting life-support systems early enough to prevent any loss of strength or general health. His program for ALS patients carries that theme of aggressiveness to its logical end. He includes everything from specific recipes for the ALS patient with a feeding tube to techniques and arguments to use in dealing with reluctant insurance companies, unenlightened doctors, and anyone else who tries to dismiss ALS patients as terminal cases. The thrust of it all is to enable ALS patients to overcome the prejudice and preconceived notions that are part of the disease's history. What Meagher is working against is "the archaic belief that all people with ALS have to die in the immediate future."

The details of Meagher's physical condition and daily routine are classic ALS details. He can move only his eyes, his mouth, his forehead, his feet (just a little bit, below the ankles), and his left leg (just enough to push a switch pad near his knee that controls his computer). He can't move anything else. He spends his waking hours reclining in a large, high-backed rocking chair securely mounted on a rolling plywood base. His hands are folded in his lap and he is usually covered with a shawl or blanket for warmth. He cannot move his head at all—it has to be propped in place, and when it falls forward or to the side, as it sometimes does, his attendant must quickly reposition it. He is 5'10" tall, although it's been ten years since he was able to stand at his full height. He weighs 110 pounds, down from a pre-ALS weight of 140. He retains control of his sphincters, so incontinence is not a problem.

One constant in Meagher's life, a critical one, is his ventilator. A compact, serious-looking piece of equipment with knobs and pressure gauges, it keeps up a steady whooshing sound that sets the rhythm of his life: it is the slow, one-two, in-out beat of a mechanical bellows; a small industrial sound, ever present; the not-so-faint sound of a factory in the distance. He is tethered to the ventilator by a plastic hose that runs to it from the tracheotomy tube protruding from his throat. On occasion, when he is out and about in a sport jacket or blazer,

Meagher covers the critical fitting at his throat with an
ascot.

Although he can move his mouth, he cannot generate
the wind he needs to make sounds; he can form the words
he wants to speak but he cannot actually speak them. He
communicates by having the nurse on duty read his lips
aloud. If they cannot make out a word, he spells it out
for them, forming each letter. When Meagher wants to
attract the attention of an attendant who is out of his line
of sight or not looking at him, he clicks his teeth together
loudly. Since no air passes through his nose or mouth
anymore, he has no sense of smell or taste.

Meagher is a handsome man with a long, angular face
set off by a thick brown mustache. It is a powerful face,
and though it lacks the full range of muscle motion, it
has remarkable range and subtlety of expression. He uses
it to add nuance to his words. Although his words are
always uttered slowly and by other, usually female,
voices, Meagher's presence is so intense he somehow
manages to overcome that and transform the voices of
others into his own voice.

Conversing with him is unique. He likes those he is
speaking with to sit directly in front of him so he can
look at them and, combined with the pace of lip reading,
it makes for a dynamic experience. Words often arrive a
letter at a time, sentences arrive one word at a time, and
each sentence is usually loaded with information and
meaning because he cannot and does not waste words.
As his thoughts and ideas come so carefully into existence in the room, it is as though he were handing you
each one, entrusting them to you. And all the time he is
talking he is looking right at you, his large brown eyes
shining with energy and experience, with his vision of
life and his knowledge of death.

Meagher rejects the idea that he possesses some extraordinary strength of will that enables him to carry on
in the face of the obstacles presented by ALS, and he has
little patience with popular portrayals of the handicapped
that present them as superhuman. "I don't think it is a
strength, or a fight," he says. "I just think it is a way to
live a normal life." Meagher has gotten beyond his body.

When asked if he feels betrayed by it, or if he has split his mind and body apart in his thinking, he says, "I believe the mind is what is human."

Meagher had his worst day with ALS early on, when he was still the only one who knew he had the disease. He doesn't go into detail about it, but he doesn't have to; he was thirty years old and terminal. He describes it simply as "one day when I really flipped out." It's become a valuable memory. "Afterwards, I thought about it and I decided it was a very unpleasant day. I was not going to be very productive or enjoy the time I had left with more days like that. If you are stuck with a bad disease which is going to give you all kinds of physical hardships, why would anybody want to force their minds into a new, unpleasant state also? There would be no reason to live if you had a bad mind and also a bad body. Why would anybody want to do that to themselves? So that was the only day I did not enjoy my mind. I could not forget it, nor do I want to forget it."

Meagher is also opposed to the existential philosophy adopted by some patients diagnosed with terminal disease. "I don't like the phrase 'I just live for today.' I believe it is definitely defeatist. I try to make plans for most of my life, not just for today. You've got to get goal-oriented." Beyond keeping himself alive and helping his patients keep themselves alive, and proving the efficacy of FSH as a treatment for ALS, Meagher's most intriguing goal is to fly around the world solo in a single-engine airplane.

"Although occasionally dormant, man's thoughts have always been in the clouds," Meagher writes in the proposal for his round-the-world project. Meagher first soloed at the age of sixteen and was an avid skydiver and glider pilot up to the time he contracted ALS. He sees his planned flight as an opportunity to raise awareness of ALS and research funds while having a hell of a good time in the bargain. In the spring of 1988 his customized airplane, a 1947 Stinson Voyager, was gradually coming together. His garage was filled with parts, and he was working with a researcher in San Francisco to develop the computer system that will enable him to fly solo with what minimal muscle control he retains. The prime elements in the computer system are electrodes that have been implanted in the back of his head, under his skull, outside the dura mater. The electrodes, placed over his visual cortex, make his eyes and his brain waves the means for operating his computer and controlling the plane. By looking at a particular section of a computer screen, Meagher can select the control function he wishes to put into operation.

The plan is enormously complicated, obviously. Not only must Meagher be able to fly the plane, he has to have systems that will handle his routine needs, like eating and tending to his ventilator, while he is aloft. He has the support of the Experimental Aviation Association and the help of his friend and neighbor Dale Majors, who has more than forty years of flying experience. Majors is realistic about the problems Meagher faces, but he's been around pilots too long to let the practical details overwhelm him. "I would be stupid to say no, he can't do it," says Majors, "because that's the history of aviation all down the line, people saying, 'He can't do it.'"

Lance Meagher is supposed to be dead, but he isn't. ALS is supposed to end his life, but it hasn't. All it's done so far is change it, and as far as he's concerned it's been a change for the better. The way he looks at it, if he hadn't gotten ALS he'd be just another typical, type-A physician, caught in the frenzy of his career. "I would never be thinking of a flight around the world," he says, speaking of a life without ALS, "I would be too busy. I would never have found a treatment, either. So I believe I have actually found a more full life than if I had not gotten ALS."

Imagine that.

VII

LANGUAGE

THE retired businessman came into the room limping slightly, his right arm hanging strangely down. He had a pleasant face, and he smiled as he was greeted by his friends. He was introduced to a visitor, and he said hello slowly and with difficulty. He took a seat and someone asked him if he wanted a cup of coffee. He smiled and said yes. He was taking part in a regular part of his day, a special coffee hour for people with a particular kind of brain damage. The visitor asked the man where he was from and the man nodded, indicating that he understood the question. Then he tried to answer, but the words would not come. He leaned forward slightly as he tried to speak, as though the words he wanted were on a shelf in his head and if he leaned forward a bit they would slide off the shelf and out of his mouth. The words did not come, but he continued to smile even as his eyes revealed his frustration and confusion. Finally, he gestured that he would be right back and left the room. Moments later he returned with a small black notebook, which he handed to the visitor. The man's name and address were written on a piece of paper that was taped inside the front cover of the notebook. The visitor read the name of the town aloud, and the man nodded and repeated the words, adding the name of the state. But the inflections and emphasis were off; the two-word name of his town and the two-word name of his state ran together in a bumpy stumble of syllables and sounds. A friend sitting next to the man repeated the words slowly and correctly for him and encouraged him to keep trying. For the next ten minutes the man patiently attempted to say the name of the town and state correctly. Again and again he tried and again and again he got it wrong.

Think about language, in the variety of its forms. The precise line of it that connects two people in serious conversation, each word selected with care, inflections modulated for accuracy. The lone point of it in the author's room at the moment of creation, when the words and sentences arrive as though they have come from some other place. The relaxed web of it at a party, language trailing about the room, supple and unpredictable, free of scrutiny and planning, in the service of simple human pleasure, language as talk, as jokes told, and secrets whispered. The murmuring bowl of it that fills stadiums and arenas when the action is slow, the low rumble of ten thousand quiet conversations, and the roaring wall of it that erupts with a score. The surprising beam of it that lights the world when the poet puts just the right words in just the right places. The slumbering mass of it stacked in the libraries, waiting to be read, language as literary enterprise, bound to outlive the writers. The silent bond of it that joins reader and book. The sudden rip of it that is a scream for help. The murderer's mumbled confession, the first-grader's correct answer, the lover's lie, the priest's blessing, the condemned man's last words, the son's promise, the professor's lecture, the madman's ranting, the President's speech, the bad novel, the dead letter, the good novel, the memo, the prayer, the chant, the baby's first coherent syllable.

There is no end to the list. Language engulfs us, swirls about us; like our bubble of oxygen, it envelops the planet. We spin it out endlessly and it comes back to us endlessly. Language is the prime mechanism for the organization and expression of the workings of the human mind, it is the skill that enables us to engage in the limitless complexities of human life, and it is the means by which we chronicle that life. Language is an elaborate, dynamic, living thing. And in most people it originates on the left side of the brain, in a few patches of cortex that, combined, are about the size of a postcard.

In the jargon of neurology, the ability to generate and comprehend language is a "higher cortical function," an extremely sophisticated type of behavior that is unique to human beings. Other special traits in the same category are creativity, personality, the ability to remember the past and plan for the future and, of course, the ability to think. All of these are products of man's highly developed cerebral cortex. They are elusive, even mysterious functions of the brain, and in thinking about them we quickly run up against all kinds of daunting questions. What is the mind? How does it work? What are the neurological underpinnings of artistic talent? What is the connection between a series of neurons firing in a certain order and the experience we know as being funny? The higher cortical functions are the human nervous system at its most advanced, and understanding the neurological and physiological principles that lie behind them provides us with what is perhaps our greatest intellectual challenge as a species. Of all the higher cortical functions, language is the one best suited to helping us meet that challenge.

Any attempt to rank the higher cortical functions in order of importance is largely subverted by the fact that a working brain blends all of them together, along with the sensory and motor functions, to establish and maintain our conscious, active existence. We are the beneficiaries of the brain's specialization and at the same time of its amazing ability to unify all of its sundry parts into a functioning whole. Nevertheless, it is possible to say that language is man's most important skill simply because without it his other special qualities remain unexpressed. Without language man is trapped inside his own head; he's like a farmer who grows the finest tomatoes in the country but doesn't have a way to ship them, so they sit in the barn and rot.

Language is the most localized of the higher cortical functions. While some specific brain structures have been associated with some kinds of memory and thought processes, those functions are anatomically much more diffuse than language. There is no single patch of cortex where long-term memory is recorded or a sole site connected with mathematical problem solving. But the parts of the brain that are involved in the various language functions are well known and have been for many years.

Language brings together all of the other functions of the brain and nervous system. It is a hybrid: part motor function, part sensory function, and part mental function. It also contains information drawn from every part of the nervous system. At the simple end, when you describe what it feels like to stub your toe, you are transforming a physical experience into language; you have linked your peripheral nervous system and your language cortex. At the more complex end of things, when you describe how you feel about the death of someone close to you, you are funneling an extraordinarily complex series of neuronal connections into your language centers as you link memories and old and new emotions with language. As you express your sadness and your happy memories and your feeling of loss and frustration in the face of death, you excite an extraordinarily complicated chain of neurons, and all that rush of information is funneled into your language centers. Of course, mere words may not prove adequate to the occasion; the experience of stubbing your toe or losing a loved one cannot be perfectly captured in language. But the important fact is that language can connect with all the disparate parts of the nervous system; the language cortex has access to all of them. This capacity for receiving input from the entire nervous system and transforming it into words and sentences is the essence of language.

Language is also unique among the higher cortical functions because it employs a system of signs, symbols, and rules that make it possible for language skills to be measured, analyzed, and evaluated objectively. Unlike IQ tests, which measure a potential for intelligent behavior, language tests can measure the actual products of the language cortex, the ability to generate and comprehend language in all of its forms. Matched up with the principle of cerebral localization, this objective, universal aspect of language takes on added importance. Careful testing, combined with an understanding of the localization of language functions, make it possible to connect specific language disorders with damage to specific parts of the cortex. While memory and thinking, like language, are universal traits, neither lends itself to such exact clinical analysis.

With language, then, we have a substantially localized higher cortical function connected to the entire nervous system, which uses a discernible system of symbols that can be measured and evaluated objectively, and which lends itself to the establishment of definite correlations between neurological disorders and their anatomic origins. What we have is an ideal model for exploring how the brain organizes itself and executes complex behavior.

The language cortex is like a keyhole connecting two oceans, the internal ocean of the mind and the external ocean of the rest of the world. The vaporous sea of ideas, memories, and thoughts that is ever roiling inside your head is made up of unuttered words and sentences and pieces of sentences. The endless waters of common reality, the waking life you share with other human beings, consist almost entirely of spoken and written words and sentences and pieces of sentences. Between the two sits the small section of the brain that gives rise to the language functions, its fleeting sparks imposing an order basic to every facet of our existence.

You were born with the capacity for language skills and you have developed them to the point where you can read, write, speak, and understand what is said to you. One day, someone you know says to you, ''Tell me about your grandmother. What was she like?'' You loved your grandmother and you think the person who asked about her is sincere, so you decide to answer. The first two sentences out of your mouth are ''My grandmother was wild. She loved parties and she made the best peach pie you ever tasted.''

This deceptively simple exchange presents almost all of the intricate steps involved in human communication.

Essentially, the use of spoken and written language involves two functions—the encoding and the decoding of information. When you speak or write you are encoding, and when you listen or read you are decoding. Now, when you were asked to talk about your grandmother, the two sentences that made up the request were dealt with first by the part of your brain responsible for registering and analyzing the sounds of spoken language. Located just above and slightly forward of your left ear, the auditory zone of the language cortex is about the size of a section of orange. This part of the brain breaks spoken words down into phonemes. The most basic units of speech, phonemes are not syllables or letters but sounds, the smallest phonetic bits, such as the *p* sound at the beginning of *pit* or the *t* sound at the end. After the auditory zone registers the various combination of sounds as words, another part of the language cortex, immediately adjacent to the auditory zone, establishes a meaning for each word. The heard words are then analyzed for their meaning in relation to each other. At the same time, inflection, tone of voice, the identity and mood of the person speaking, the circumstances at the time of the conversation, and other modifying factors are taken into account. As an example of the role of the latter two factors, if the person who asked you about your grandmother was not a friend but a detective who suspects your grandmother was a bank robber, your response to the identical sentences would likely be very different.

Decoding, then, consists of three elements: the analysis of the sound involves phonology, the analysis of the individual words involves semantics, and the analysis of the sentence structure involves syntax. Though there are many theories about how the brain decodes speech, some very fundamental details remain unknown. It simply isn't possible to say, for instance, exactly how the language cortex distinguishes between a verb and a noun.

Still, there has to be a capacity for remembering vocabulary, a mental dictionary that can be tapped when a word comes in via the auditory language zone. But recognizing a word and associating it with its correct meaning are two different things. This point is illustrated by

the key word in the first sentence your friend uses—
grandmother. *Grandmother* can be associated with at
least three different definitions: the literal definition is the
mother of a parent, the generic definition might be a nice
old lady with gray hair and lots of grandchildren, and the
specific definition is the mother of one of *your* parents.
You knew which definition your friend was referring to
because he prefaced the word *grandmother* with the word
your. But your brain recognized the word *grandmother*
before it analyzed the sentence's syntax and selected the
correct meaning of the word as dictated by the word *your*.

Of all the words in the two sentences of the statement,
grandmother is the one that requires the most complex
analysis, the one that calls up the most elaborate collection of associations. The other words are fairly clear and
simple. *Tell* is a verb, *me* refers to the speaker, *about* is
a preposition that leaves the topic wide open, and *your*
modifies *grandmother*. Understanding those words sep-
arately and as a group is routine for the language cortex.
Dealing with *grandmother* is something else again, because once you realize the word refers to your grandmother, a flood of memories, ideas, and even emotions
is released. And now we are moving beyond the limits
of the language cortex in the decoding process and bringing in other parts of the brain, including the frontal lobes,
which are believed to play a part in the analysis of complex language, and the many structures connected with
memory and emotion. The word *grandmother* in this
context may have triggered a literal picture in your mind
of your grandmother sipping a drink and laughing at a
party. And that image may have been followed instantly
by one of you sitting in her kitchen and eating a piece of
her peach pie, an image so strong you could even remember how the pie tasted. (Remembering how something
tasted and then describing it is a multi-faceted neurological performance.)

While relatively little is known about how the brain
analyzes phonology, semantics, and syntax, while also
figuring in things like inflection and tone, we do know
that a specific patch of cortex is responsible for ''comprehension.'' Known as Wernicke's area, after Carl Wer-

nicke, the German neuropsychiatrist who first established
its location and role in language functions in 1874, this
encompasses a small, triangular section of cortex just
behind the auditory language zone at the back of the left
temporal lobe (above and forward of your left ear). Wernicke's area is responsible for determining the meaning
of spoken and written language, as well as providing the
first step in the production of comprehensible language
when speaking or writing. It is here that in the decoding
process the rules of semantics and syntax are applied.

The comprehension of spoken language depends on the
brain's ability to deal with all kinds of subtle details. It
must be able to recognize verbs, nouns, adjectives, ad-
verbs, conjunctions, and even articles and to parse out
their various influences on the meaning of a statement.
And the order of the words plays an important role in the
decoding of language as well. This detail is illustrated by
the second sentence that your friend used, ''What was
she like?'' To change the meaning and tone of that statement all you have to do is move the word *like* from the
end to the beginning of the sentence, and you have a
slangy, 1960s type of inquiry into her political, racial,
or religious background: ''Like, what was she?'' In longer
chunks of speech, decoding requires that the brain remembers ever more complicated strings of words in their proper
order. While this seems simple enough, it entails a specialized kind of short-term memory that is crucial for language comprehension.

Tone of voice also plays an important role in decoding.
If we switch examples for just a moment, it's possible to
see how tone of voice can make a sentence mean the
exact opposite of what the actual words in the sentence
mean. You run into a friend who has just been given a
raise and a promotion and you ask him how he's doing.
He says, ''I'm just great,'' and you know he really means
it. A little while later you run into another friend, who
has just been fired. You ask him how he's doing and he
says the exact same thing, but by the way he says it you
know the guy is miserable. Exactly how the brain makes
these kinds of distinctions is not known, but it seems
clear that it is a skill that draws on more than the lan-

guage cortex. The ability to recognize and understand a mood factor in speech could be the result of a link between the language cortex and the parts of the listener's brain that are involved in mood. That is to say, the interpretation of tone of voice is likely made possible by cortical connections that add emotional and psychological elements to the language comprehension function.

And so, as you continue to scan the mental manifestations of the word *grandmother*—image after image, memory after memory you begin to formulate what you are going to say about her, and in so doing you slip imperceptibly from the act of decoding to the act of encoding. According to A. R. Luria, the famous twentieth-century Soviet psychologist and neuropsychological researcher, the first step in any conscious activity is intention. In this instance, you intended to listen to your friend and now you intend to answer him. This would seem so fundamental and obvious as to not bear mentioning, but it's important because Luria attributes this crucial function to the frontal lobes. Which means that all language activity depends on a precondition that originates in the frontal lobes. And that detail serves to illustrate the built-in limits of the concept of cerebral localization. You can fire up your language centers in the left temporal region only after the spark of intention is struck just behind your forehead.

With the intention to answer, you proceed to execute a response by triggering the encoding mechanisms. You have to translate into words and sentences and say aloud the various ideas and images that were prompted by mention of "your grandmother." Eliminating everything but the subject at hand from the encoding system is essential in this process. A preliminary encoding function enables us to select only the things we wish to put into language at any given moment and to suppress everything else: alternative definitions of words you are going to use and any other thoughts you might have in your head at the time as well. You won't respond to your friend by commenting on the weather or a baseball game you saw the night before. Somehow, only your grandmother information is processed by Wernicke's area.

Basically, the decoding and encoding processes are two sides of the same coin. When you decode, Wernicke's area breaks down spoken sentences and comprehends their meaning. When you encode, or produce language, Wernicke's area builds sentences that make sense, transforming your images of your grandmother into proper sentences according to the rules of semantics and syntax. As is the case with the role of Wernicke's area in decoding, it is unclear exactly how these rules are applied in encoding. Some researchers believe that so-called Freudian slips are evidence that, in the act of encoding, the brain first assembles a framework for a sentence and then plugs in the appropriate words. The brain knows that an understandable sentence requires certain types of words—a subject, a verb, and an object, for instance. So, when producing speech, it first plans the basic form of the sentence and then searches the mental dictionary for the correct words. According to this model, a Freudian slip occurs when the wrong word of a particular type is slipped into the slot in the sentence created for that type of word. When you say "I hate my job" but you mean to say "I love my job," you have slipped the wrong word into the verb slot.

Your images of your grandmother are fed into Wernicke's area, where the sentences you want to say are generated. That information is then transferred to another part of the language cortex, called Broca's area, which is the part of the brain responsible for the motor aspect of language production. Named after Pierre-Paul Broca, the French surgeon and anthropologist who established its role in language functions in 1861, Broca's area is a little larger than a quarter and is located on the side of the left frontal lobe slightly higher and just a couple of inches forward of Wernicke's area. These two main language centers are connected by the arcuate fasciculus, a large bundle of nerve fibers that runs in a tight arc beneath the cortex from Wernicke's area to Broca's area. Broca's area receives input from Wernicke's area, then transforms it, and forwards a program to the motor cortex for the execution of the movements that will result in the correct vocalization of the sentences, complete with proper inflections and tone of voice.

Once Broca's area activates the motor cortex, the words are spoken and the cycle of human communication is complete—you heard what your friend said, you understood, you responded, and he heard and understood your response. Your response—"My grandmother was wild. She loved parties and she made the best peach pie you ever tasted"—was sufficiently provocative to start a long and pleasant conversation about your wild grandmother, *wild* and *grandmother* being two words not usually connected.

One way to grasp the workings of the language cortex and to truly appreciate the speed at which they are executed is simply to remember what it was like the first time you studied a foreign language. Recall the torturous experience of producing a complete sentence, how the language process ground to a halt as you struggled to remember where in the sentence the verb was supposed to go. Recall those long, deadly afternoons in the language lab, sitting there with earphones on, staring straight ahead, while a strange voice droned on and your scrambled brain strained to break up the meaningless flow of sounds and transform it into what you knew was really a simple statement about a man and his umbrella. Recall the old joke about French being a simple language, so simple that in France even little kids speak it. Recall your relief when you reached that point in your education where the choice of classes was left up to you, and how foreign languages were summarily banned from all future curricula. What all you failed students of French, Spanish, and (bless you) Latin can draw from those dusty memories is the simple lesson that language is based on very exacting rules, and that the ability to use language well and quickly necessarily depends on a capacity for applying those rules instantly, constantly, and efficiently. And that capacity is the province of the language cortex.

There is no question that language is bound up with things like emotion, personality, and state of mind. And as we attempt to sketch out possible connections between the language cortex and different parts of the brain, it's

important to keep in mind that the language functions
are part of an integrated, whole thing that is an individual
person. Basically, what we are trying to do is somewhat
similar to an attempt to determine the layout of a city's
subway system by flying over the city and studying the
flow and movements of the population. It's easy to forget
that the city is a functioning whole if you are trying to
look through it and imagine the grids that lie beneath its
streets. That is one of the main problems when you speculate about the workings of the higher cortical functions.
In a sense, the human brain is two very different things
at once: an elaborate arrangement of neurons, a physiological thing that works according to the basic and known
rules of biochemistry, and a metaphysical mystery capable of behavior beyond all understanding. Any attempt
to understand any single part or function of the brain will
suffer if the big picture isn't kept in focus at all times.
As we shall see, when it comes to language the key to
keeping that focus is old and familiar. It is in the clinical
setting of a rehabilitation hospital, in the speech pathology department, that the endless personal nuances of
language function are best seen and best understood.

Most of what we know about the neurological foun-
dations of the language functions has been learned by
studying and testing people with brain damage, and in
most cases the brain damage has been caused by a stroke.
This is the traditional clinical method of medical research, in which the nature of the normal function is
determined by the exploration of the abnormal function.
Broca's initial proposal about the localization of language function was the result of autopsies performed on
patients who had exhibited language disorders. One of
those patients was a man in his forties who was given the
nickname Tan because the only thing he could say was
"tan, tan," although he was able to understand language
and communicate by gestures. When Broca examined
Tan's brain he found a lesion that encompassed what we
now call Broca's area and he deduced that area's role in
language production. Wernicke's localization of a language comprehension zone resulted from similar meth-

ods. Today, research into the language functions and the neuroanatomy of language follows that same basic pattern, aided and improved greatly by sophisticated testing that defines the nature and limits of the language disorders in great detail, and by advanced imaging techniques, which reveal the exact location and extent of the underlying damage to the brain.

Disorders of language function are called aphasia. The two main types of aphasia correspond to the two main parts of the language cortex.

Broca's aphasia, also known as motor aphasia, is a disorder caused by damage to Broca's area. A person with Broca's aphasia can understand spoken and written language but cannot produce normal speech and cannot write. In severe cases, there may be no words forthcoming; in less severe cases, speech will be halting, the words coming slowly and, to varying degrees, not very clearly. People with Broca's aphasia tend to eliminate articles, conjunctions, and prepositions from their speech and usually produce fewer than twenty words in a minute. The sentence "We went to the baseball game and had a good time," if spoken by a Broca's aphasic, might come out along the lines of "We . . . went . . . ball . . . game . . . good . . . time. . . ." Besides missing words, the sentence would lack normal rhythm. The gist of the sentence would be preserved, making a primitive kind of communication possible. But it isn't a very satisfying kind of communication, and a critical factor in Broca's aphasia is the afflicted person's painful and possibly psychologically damaging awareness of his deficit.

A Broca's aphasic knows what he wants to say, but he can't say it because the part of his brain that transforms his conceived words into spoken words is damaged. He has the content but not the form. A Wernicke's aphasic, on the other hand, has the form but not the content. He can produce plenty of properly modulated speech, but it is meaningless because Wernicke's area, the part of the brain that generates comprehensible language, is damaged. The speech of a Wernicke's aphasic is a normal-sounding flow of nonsense in which words are strung together with no regard to their meaning. In fact, some of the words may not be words at all but totally bogus wordlike things constructed out of various sounds and syllables. And not only is a Wernicke's aphasic unable to produce any language with meaning, he is unable to understand any language that he hears, and he can't read. For all practical purposes, Wernicke's aphasia destroys all communication. The Wernicke's aphasic is completely cut off from the world and eerily oblivious of that fact.

There are several other aphasias. Global aphasia, which involves the loss of all language functions, is the same as Wernicke's in that the person is unable to comprehend any language and unable to produce any with meaning. Global aphasics, however, are unable to produce the fluent babble of a Wernicke's aphasic, because they also have damage to Broca's area.

Conduction aphasia, caused by a lesion in the arcuate fasciculus, cuts off the flow of nerve impulses between Wernicke's area and Broca's area, while leaving both intact. Conduction aphasics can comprehend spoken and written language but because there is an interruption of the flow from Wernicke's to Broca's area, their speech, while fluent, is meaningless. An irony of conduction aphasia is the fact that conduction aphasics can hear their own speech and are aware of the fact that it is incomprehensible. Like Broca's aphasics, they know something is wrong with them. In addition, there are other, rarer aphasias, caused by lesions in different parts of the language cortex that in effect eliminate specific aspects of language function. Pure word deafness, in which language functions are normal except for an inability to understand spoken language, is one of these.

For Dr. Martha Taylor Sarno, head of the speech pathology department at the Howard A. Rusk Institute of Rehabilitation Medicine in Manhattan, the systems for classifying the various types of aphasia are useful tools that ultimately miss the point. As far as Dr. Sarno is concerned, there are many different kinds of aphasia as there are aphasia patients. "I think language is uniquely individual. Each of us has our own universe of language, our own way of communicating that is uniquely personal.

Language *is* part of the personality. And that's the problem with aphasia—once language is damaged, one's sense of self is devastated. All of a sudden, your self-image is something else, you're a different person. And the patient will describe to you, if he can, that he feels so altered; that he knows that his means of controlling his environment, which is his verbal skill, is no longer available to him.''

It is the social and psychological aspects of aphasia, as opposed to the anatomical and physiological, that most interest and concern Sarno. At any given time, she and her staff of seven speech pathologists have between sixty and a hundred patients under their care, and while the exact cause of each patient's language disorder is an important detail, it is the effect of that disorder on the patient's life that must be dealt with. In fact, it's the only thing that really can be dealt with. Aside from making a diagnosis, directing the acute care, and seeking to prevent future stroke, a neurologist can't do much for a patient with aphasia except pass him or her along to a speech pathologist. So, while each patient who enters Sarno's service is initially evaluated, and the aphasia is classified by type, that is merely the beginning. Though the speech pathologist's primary job is to work to improve the speech and language skills of the patients, there is a lot more to it than that.

The Rusk Institute occupies a small corner of the world, hard by the East River at the very end of East Thirty-fourth Street, at the windy edge of Manhattan, next door to a busy commercial helicopter pad. It sits on the northern end of the sprawling New York University Medical Center, which stretches along First Avenue for five blocks in a complex that includes the NYU School of Medicine and the city morgue. People with every conceivable physical handicap receive rehabilitation treatment at Rusk. Rusk has an atmosphere of remarkable energy and busyness; great things happen there every day. It is an inspirational place, not in a corny, "Theme from *Rocky*" way, but in the genuine way it inspires anyone who enters it, even on a visit, to do their best at what they are doing. A lot of serious, hardworking people are

engaged in a lot of serious hard work as the patients and
their families confront and learn to live with some very
harsh realities. Just walking the halls and riding the elevators is an overwhelming experience. There are para-
plegics, quadriplegics, people with one leg, people with
no legs, people with no hands, stroke victims, accident
victims, victims of fate, if there is such a thing. There
are people of every race and every age. (A strong young
man with powerful arms rolls by in a wheelchair, his
girlfriend by his side.) On one floor there is a display
case filled with different kinds of artificial limbs—hard,
bloodless replicas of arms and legs, hands and feet, constructed of gleaming metal and flesh-colored plastic. The
Rusk Institute is not an easy place in which to be, but
you can't fight it, even if you're just passing through.
When you are in the building you have to drop your discomfort and guilt, and let the reality of the place take
you. What is going on there requires respect.

Surrounded by patients with every kind of physical
handicap, the aphasics also have a physical manifestation
of the insult to their brains. A stroke that affects the language centers on the left side of the brain often affects
the parts of the brain that control the right side of the
body. The degree of paresis varies from case to case and
usually improves over time. Recently afflicted patients
may be confined to wheelchairs, those who are further
along may be using crutches or canes, and the most advanced can often walk unaided or with the help of a brace.
Aphasics also often wear braces to support the right arm.
Physical therapy is a regular part of their treatment reg-
imen.

It quickly becomes apparent at Rusk how different
aphasia is from even the worst kind of physical disability.
Waiting for an elevator, for instance, one can easily strike
up a conversation with a patient who has a strictly physical handicap—slow elevators are a good subject to start
with. That kind of basic social behavior makes for a relaxed atmosphere that in turn helps everybody keep things
in perspective. But you can't make easy small talk with
an aphasic. And there are no prosthetic devices available
to them to help alleviate their handicap.

A motor language aphasia can affect a person's self-image, Sarno points out, because the aphasics can hear themselves speak. "But when the language itself is impaired," she says, "when the nouns are in the wrong places and when the prepositions are gone and when the sentence hasn't got any anatomy, then the patient can really feel like a stupid idiot. And he'll tell you he feels dumb. I mean, it's no accident that the word *dumb* is used to describe speechlessness."

A great number of aphasic patients are aware of their disorder. "They are acutely aware of being grossly different, in a sense dehumanized," Sarno says. "What's more human than speaking? It's the one thing that differentiates us from the other animal species. And it is such a biologically determined behavior it's totally programmed in. It isn't something you learn, it just happens, as long as you have a normal sensory system. To have that taken away, or reduced in any way, is far worse than any other disability that a person could possibly have."

Twice each weekday, at 10:00 A.M. and again at 1:00 P.M., new patients are tested in a small soundproof room. The room is just large enough to hold a filing cabinet and a small table and chair. During the testing the patient and the speech pathologist face each other across the table. The patient is usually in a wheelchair outfitted with a special attachment on which to rest his weakened right arm. Because Rusk is strictly a rehabilitation hospital, the aphasia patients arrive from other hospitals. So they are usually two to three weeks beyond their strokes when they are initially evaluated at Rusk.

For this session, the patient is a stunningly healthy-looking man of seventy-seven. He is a big guy with large arms and a sunburnt face who has clearly spent a lot of time working outdoors. He is wearing a red, short-sleeved sweatshirt and matching red sweatpants. He has a fringe of curly white hair. He barely fits in his wheelchair, and is clearly uncomfortable with the entire situation. He has had a stroke twenty-three days earlier, but the only evidence that anything is wrong with him is the wheelchair and the way his right arm rests limply upon it.

The speech pathologist begins by asking the man where

he lives. She names the boroughs, starting with Manhattan, and he responds to each with a firm but indistinct "no" until she says "Queens?", and then he says a quiet "Yeah."

"Where in Queens do you live?" she then asks. He responds with a mumbled phrase that contains a very rough version of the word *Queens* and a second sound with a *z* in it.

The speech pathologist says, "Queens Plaza?" and the man nods and repeats the words, which are much clearer in repetition than they were when he said them the first time.

Then, detecting an accent in his garbled speech, the pathologist says, "You have an accent. Can you tell me where you were born?" He understands what she says but he can't initiate an answer, so she again asks him a series of questions.

"Were you born in the United States?" she asks. Again, he responds with a firm but indistinct "No."

"Where were you born?" she asks. He answers with a low mumble of sounds, and at the end of it the speech pathologist picks out the words *another country* and repeats them, to which the man says, "Yeah."

"Were you born in Germany?" she asks, and his "No" is the firmest and clearest yet.

"Italy?" she says, and he answers with another indistinct "Yeah."

"Where in Italy?" she asks, and he says something long and completely unintelligible. His speaking has a loose quality to it when it extends for more than a syllable or two; the sounds spill out in a jumble, soft and blurry.

Next, the speech pathologist draws a rough sketch of Italy and asks the man to point to the part of it where he was born. "Were you born in the country or in a town?" she asks. And she continues the casual conversation, asking him about his wife and family. The brief, pretest exchange reveals the man to be oriented and able to comprehend simple spoken language. He is able to follow the questions, even when they consist only of a single, inflected word, and he always attempts an answer.

The battery of tests the speech pathologist administers measures everything from the patient's ability to move his lips to his ability to write a narrative describing the action taking place in a specially prepared drawing. After checking the man's oral agility by having him purse his lips, open and close his mouth, stick out his tongue, and so on, the speech pathologist takes out two trays of objects and has the man name them. The objects in the first tray are a comb, a ring, a key, a cup, an ashtray, a thimble, a padlock, and a large paper clip. The second tray contains a knife, a fork, a bottle, a shoelace, a brush, a jar, a bottle opener, and tweezers. The man does pretty well with this; his single-syllable words are easy to understand, though he leaves the *ash* out of *ashtray* and is stumped by the thimble. In the next test, the man is supposed to describe the uses of some more objects, including a toy gun, a screwdriver, a sponge, a clock, and a razor. The test is designed to measure his ability to use words, and though the man seems to recognize the objects and understand the test, he does less well. Shown the toy gun, he first says "Gun" and then, when the speech pathologist asks him what it's for, he says, "Shoot." As the test proceeds, a pattern develops in which the man says the name of the object and then, when asked what it is for, produces garbled noise that may or may not contain a relevant word. Handed the object in question, he will act out its proper use, turning the screwdriver, for instance, and saying the word *screw*. The man knows he is not doing well on this test and gradually he becomes visibly frustrated, shaking his head and making a face.

Arrayed in the trays, the common articles used for these tests look like junk culled from some bottomless kitchen drawer. But as the man holds them in his good left hand and struggles to name them and describe their uses, the objects take on added meaning. His concentration transforms them from the mundane into strangely powerful symbols of the world as it was before his stroke, when he paid no attention to such trivial items, just as he paid no attention to his ability to speak. In that room, over time, a sadness has collected around those objects as they have gone unnamed, misnamed, or clumsily named by patient after patient. A shoelace, a thimble, a cup, a key. They are such plain things, and yet, in the absence of words to describe them, they are such moving things.

As the session continues, the tests become more and more difficult, and the gravity of the man's aphasia becomes increasingly apparent. In a sentence repetition test, he is supposed to repeat a series of sentences, the first of which is the single word "Look," and the last of which is "Riding his black horse, the general came to the scene of the battle and began shouting at his brave men." Through the first eight sentences the man does okay, though his words are very slurred. Then, on number nine—"The sun was shining throughout the day"—he gets the words *sun shining* and then drifts into an unintelligible mumble. He is also unable to generate lists of words that begin with the letters *f, a,* and *s.* He is unable to describe a picture that the speech therapist shows him, a drawing of some children who are trying to steal cookies while their mother is washing dishes. The only thing he does well on for the rest of the session is a comprehension test that requires him to answer yes or no to a series of simple, somewhat odd questions. "Are you a man?" "Do you eat a banana before you peel it?" "Does it snow in July?" and "Do you cut the grass with an ax?" are among them. As the session ends, the man begins to weep quietly. The speech therapist gives him a tissue and comforts him, speaking softly to him as he wipes his eyes. For all practical purposes he is not able to produce intelligible speech. The speech pathologist later explains that the man has "a fairly severe nonfluent aphasia," but even that is an improvement from when she briefly saw him earlier, closer to his stroke.

"It's a real therapeutic relationship," Sarno says of the patient-speech pathologist connection. "Very private, very, very close. It's a one-on-one kind of thing which might last for many months or even years. And the thrust of the relationship focuses on how the patient feels at different stages and how he's recovering."

"If it wasn't for the Rusk Institute I would have been

up the creek at the age of thirty-four,'' says Grace Bradley, who had a stroke in 1966 that wiped out her ability to speak. Now fifty-seven, Grace works as a volunteer at Rusk. "I had my stroke on a Monday, in the middle of the night. I had terrible crazy things in my head, and I fell down. I went into a semi-coma.'' At the time of the stroke, her son was nine and her daughter was six. Grace recalls that her daughter asked if it could happen to her, too.

Grace had her stroke at the end of August and spent three weeks in a Manhattan hospital before transferring to Rusk, where she spent one month as an inpatient and was then an outpatient until May 1967.

Upon waking from her coma, Grace could understand what was said to her, she could read, she could repeat some words, but she couldn't speak spontaneously. Her right side was paralyzed—"completely gone,'' she says. She was devastated, terrified, embarrassed. She remembered that time was sometimes confused at the beginning; she wasn't sure if the doctors were coming in the morning, the afternoon, or the evening. When she watched television, a half-hour show "seemed like half a day.'' Her comprehension was intact and she knew the sentences she wanted to say, but she couldn't produce them. To this day, she still "sees'' what she wants to say. "I can visualize in my brain, or in my forehead, what words I want to say, but I can't . . .''

She can't always say them. More than twenty years later, Grace still has a language deficit. She speaks well and clearly, but slowly. There is some hesitation, a slight halting, and close listening reveals small cracks in her speech. She will sometimes switch small words—*was* for *is*—or leave them out altogether. She will get the tense wrong or mix up plurals and singulars. "The insurance don't covered going home.'' "When week was over.'' "The only thing it's fearing is fear itself.'' These kinds of sentences pop up irregularly in her conversation, and most of her usage is correct. Over the course of a long conversation, the great majority of her sentences are properly constructed, but there is a fragile feeling to her conversations, and the occasional lapses confirm the impression that speaking requires extra effort and concentration for Grace. She is really putting her words together when she speaks, and it isn't always easy for her.

Grace is fully conscious of her limits. "Abstract speech is difficult for me," she says. This includes her comprehension as well as her production of language. If a conversation becomes too complicated in form—if, for instance, it loops back on itself, and she is asked suddenly to refer back to an earlier exchange—she can't always follow the thought. It is as if she deals with language in a straightforward, linear form. Nuances and complexities, in structure or in meaning, are difficult for her to grasp. In fact, she is so tuned in to the rhythm of speech and her own abilities that she can anticipate problems in a conversation before they occur. And when she uses the wrong word, she knows.

Part of the problem, she says, is nervousness. "When you're tense, you're nothing," she says, "you can't do anything. When you relax, you can." This is a key point for Grace. She sees the connection between her language skills and her general state of being, and she knows they affect each other. She sums it up neatly—"I think the whole body and the speech comes together."

If Grace still has problems so many years after her stroke, she is also still recovering. "Recently, I was able to make innuendos. Before I was only able to think about it." That kind of subtle progress excites Grace. She also remembers unexpectedly running into some people she knew and making small talk. She couldn't wait to tell her husband about it. "I was absolutely amazed. I had bantered."

Grace, who has a distinct limp and wears a brace on her right forearm, waited ten years before returning to Rusk as a volunteer because the memories were too strong; the experience had been so intense. "I think I'm serving a good purpose here," she says. "I don't tell everybody, 'Hey, look at me, I had a stroke.' I tell a few patients, depressed patients. They come in here so lost."

VIII

THOUGHT

An exploration of the disorders of the human nervous system inevitably leads to the smoky border between neurology and psychology, that mysterious territory where the least understood parts of the brain give rise to the most complex human traits. Mood, emotion, drive, a sense of self, a sense of the world, a sense of self in relation to the world, and all the other components of daily reality originate in nervous tissue. This thing called love is a biochemical phenomenon, as are all the thoughts and feelings human beings experience. They are the products of neurotransmitters—the chemical agents that neurons use to communicate with each other—and the chains of neurons the transmitters link together.

Like moving and speaking, the ability to control one's thoughts is a nervous system function so basic to normal life that few people ever think about it. It is the good fortune of the great majority of human beings that they are able to order their thoughts and ideas in a way that allows them to take part successfully in the routine course of human events. Without conscious effort, they make sense of the constant stream of information flowing in from the world around them and carry out the countless tasks that constitute a typical day—they wash and clothe and feed themselves, they go to work and to school, they participate in family and community life—because their nervous systems are anatomically and biochemically nor-

174

mal. They are wired for living, and because the wiring is intact they live in a recognizable world and experience a reality whose essential elements are common. They are able to function in society because, in a sense, they all think alike.

For those afflicted with schizophrenia, however, the blessing of ordered thought is lacking. Thinking is a diffuse, whole-brain activity that involves a number of different functions, including memory, language, the application of intellect, and the processing of sensory information. The range of activities that can be classified as thinking is broad—a composer thinks as he composes a symphony, and a truck driver thinks as he maneuvers through traffic. In spite of the many different kinds of thinking man is capable of, however, there are fundamental elements common to all human thought, certain mental processes by which the mind organizes itself for thinking and then thinks. Because schizophrenia is a disorder in which these basic elements of thought are disturbed, schizophrenics experience a world profoundly different from the one the rest of us know. Because of organic differences in their brains, their world is an extraordinary version of ours, a strange and frightening place where the rules that normally govern the workings of the human mind do not apply.

Schizophrenics suffer auditory hallucinations, bizarre delusions, and a phenomenon known as thought insertion, among other symptoms. The voices they hear may be God's, the devil's, or a benign commentator's. Their delusions typically involve elaborate conspiracies in which they are being watched by some government agency or even by aliens from other planets. They sometimes describe how thoughts that are not their own are inserted into their heads, or their own thoughts are stolen from them by outside forces. In addition, schizophrenic thought is characterized by a number of distinguishable disorders of structure and content.

Schizophrenics often demonstrate ''loose association'' and string ideas together with little regard for sense. Seemingly overwhelmed by thoughts and sensations, the schizophrenic mind cannot draw any ordered or logical statements out of the jumble. A classic example: "My last teacher in that subject was Professor A. He was a man with black eyes. There are also blue and gray eyes and other sorts too. I have heard it said that snakes have green eyes. All people have eyes." One patient was prompted thus: "Why don't you tell me a little bit about what you think about current political issues, like the energy crisis, for example." The response makes it clear that the patient knew what the subject was—the energy crisis—but was not able to make sense of the ideas, images, and memories the phrase triggered. "They're destroying too many cattle and oil just to make soap," he replied. "If we need soap when you can jump into a pool of water and then when you go to buy your gasoline, m-my folks always thought they should, get pop but the best thing to get, is motor oil and money. May as well go there and trade in some, pop caps and, uh, tires, and tractors to grup, car garages, so they can pull cars away from wrecks, is what I believed in."

Schizophrenia, which primarily strikes young adults in their late teens and early twenties, afflicts one percent of the world population, regardless of ethnic or cultural background. It is estimated that as many as twenty million people in the world have schizophrenia. In the United States, two to three million people have the disease, and there are 100,000 to 200,000 new cases each year. There are more schizophrenics in American mental hospitals—300,000 of them fill about half the beds—than patients with any other single disease. Beyond the suffering of the individuals with the disease, schizophrenia exacts an extra-heavy toll on society because it attacks young people just as they are assuming their responsible roles in life. The estimated costs of the disease in medical expenses, social services and lost productivity range from $20 billion to $48 billion per year in the United States alone. The cost in suffering to the victims, their families, and their friends cannot be estimated, nor can the impact of the disease on daily life in American streets, where thousands of schizophrenics wander untreated, ranting and homeless. One expert on the disease puts the number of schizophrenics living in public shelters and on the streets at 150,000.

Schizophrenia was first identified at the turn of the century by Emil Kraepelin, a German neuropsychiatrist who called it "dementia praecox" because of the precocious deterioration of the intellect that characterizes the disease. The term *schizophrenia* was first used to describe the condition by Eugen Bleuler, a Swiss psychiatrist of the same era who, along with Kraepelin, is credited with establishing it as a distinct disorder. Unfortunately, the term *schizophrenia*, with the prefix *schizo* meaning "split," has come to be widely misunderstood by the general public as referring to a dual-personality syndrome. Schizophrenics do not have the dual personality that people think of and refer to as a split personality. The split that Bleuler was referring to was between his patients' ideas and their emotions, between their intellects and their affects. Hence, a schizophrenic might laugh at bad news or cry at good news, to use simple examples.

Generally recognized as a chronic, progressive disease, schizophrenia's course is marked by flare-ups and remissions. In terms of prognosis, the "rule of thirds" applies to schizophrenia. One third of the patients will recover enough to hold jobs, have relationships, and generally function in society, though usually at a reduced level. One third will wind up at the other end of the spectrum, completely cut off from normal roles in society, the kind of worst cases that fifty years ago would have been chronically hospitalized. The other third falls in between, unable to function in any normal capacity but not as far gone as the worst cases.

The evolution of our knowledge of schizophrenia and its treatments over the last fifty years epitomize broader changes in the approach to mental illness. Today, schizophrenia is recognized as a brain disorder, with its roots in biochemical and, possibly, anatomic abnormalities. In the years before the organic concept of mental illness became dominant, schizophrenia was believed to be a "functional" disorder—as opposed to organic—in which the family and environment, particularly the patient's relationship with his or her mother, was the critical element. (That old idea seems particularly ironic in light of the fact that one of the most important features of schizophrenia as we understand it today is a strong genetic factor. While the incidence of the disease among the general population is one percent, among family members of schizophrenics it is 15 percent.) Schizophrenics have never been well served by medicine; the disease is too complex, too baffling. Even today, while the emphasis on research into the underlying causes of schizophrenia is exciting, it can be read as a de facto acknowledgment that current treatments are less than successful. And they are. But before we look at those treatments, and at the research, we have to look at what preceded them; only then can we appreciate how far we have come, and how far we have to go. As UCLA psychiatrist and schizophrenia researcher Dr. Arnold Scheibel put it, when asked to describe the progress made in the last fifty years, "It's an ascent, from abysmal ignorance to still quite complete ignorance."

Of all the strange and unnatural acts man has engaged in over the course of time, one of the strangest and most unnatural was psychosurgery as it was practiced in the quarter century between 1935 and 1960. A brutal procedure born of ignorances, arrogance, and expediency, the frontal lobotomy was nothing less than an attempt to "operate" on the minds of the mentally ill. More than 30,000 psychosurgical procedures were performed in the United States during those years, and in every single case the basic rules of surgery were violated because no surgeon who performed such an operation knew enough about what he was doing to justify his action. The operations were mutilating stabs in the dark; most of the time the surgeons couldn't even see the brain tissue they were cutting because they operated through such small openings in the skull. But that didn't matter, because it wasn't the brain they were really operating on anyway. They were operating on the thinking process itself, and on the personality. As explained in a major textbook on the subject published in 1950, at the height of psychosurgery's popularity, the objective was to alter the behavior of chronically ill, institutionalized patients, restoring them to "effective citizenship" and returning them to the community. "In other cases," the authors candidly continued, "even though the patients must remain in the hospital, they are relieved of their terrific suicidal and homicidal drives and there is a gratifying reduction in the wear and tear on hospital equipment and personnel."

In a frontal lobotomy, also known as a leucotomy (from *leuco*, Greek for "white"), the surgeon destroyed white matter in both the left and right frontal lobes in a manner analogous to coring an apple. The operation interrupted neuronal pathways connecting the frontal lobes with the limbic system and other parts of the brain. A collection of linked structures located near the center of the brain, the little understood, extraordinarily complex limbic system is known to play a critical role in emotional states and behavior. The desired result of the surgery was a flattening of affect that rendered previously agitated or uncontrollable persons docile. Unfortunately, there was no way to know what the results of any given operation might be. While thousands of psychosurgical procedures "worked," thousands more did not, leaving already mentally disturbed patients with what amounted to traumatic brain damage. For all practical purposes, those patients for whom psychosurgery provided no relief for their diagnosed mental disorders may as well have been hit in the head with an ax, albeit a small, sterile one.

Although one might assume that such radical surgery came into common practice only after years of research and experimentation, the psychosurgery era was primarily the result of one man's enthusiastic response to a single report about work done on two trained chimpanzees. The man was António Egas Moniz, the father of psychosurgery. In the summer of 1935, Moniz, a Portuguese neurologist who had already made a major contribution to his field by developing a technique for cerebral angiography, attended the Second International Neurological Congress in London. The paper that inspired Moniz detailed a series of experiments, by Carlyle Jacobsen, in which it was shown that anxiety and neurotic states could not be induced in primates whose frontal lobes had been removed. Prior to surgery, the animals had been taught to perform certain tasks and had been conditioned to expect certain results. When the researchers arranged it so the monkeys made mistakes, the intact animals became upset, frustrated, and angry. Under the same conditions but without their frontal lobes, the animals remained calm when they made mistakes. Moniz approached one of the authors of the paper and proposed performing a similar operation on disturbed humans. He was rebuffed. Undeterred, he returned to Portugal, hooked up with a willing neurosurgeon, and went to work. Moniz directed his first psychosurgical procedure on a human on November 12, 1935, just months after the London conference.

Before Moniz, there had been a few scattered cases of brain surgery aimed at modifying disturbed behavior in humans. In the 1880s, Gottlieb Burckhardt, who ran a small mental hospital in Switzerland, had operated on six of his patients. His work was incredibly brash, considering how primitive the concept of cerebral localization and neurosurgical techniques were at that time. His idea was to eliminate specific symptoms of psychoses by removing portions of the brain related to the symptoms. He operated on one patient four different times, removing pieces of her brain from four locations. In a classic example of accumulating facts to justify bad science, Burckhardt carefully weighed the chunks of brain after he removed them. He reported that all of his patients showed some improvement. In 1910, the Estonian surgeon, Lodivicus Puusepp performed three psychosurgical procedures but was not satisfied with his results and did not pursue the matter.

Moniz's underlying theory of mental illness was as extraordinary as his lack of research. He believed that mental disorders were caused by certain fixed patterns of neurons in the brain, particularly in the frontal lobes. These fixed patterns of neurons generated fixed patterns of disturbed thought and behavior. Moniz's solution to the problem was to surgically destroy these ''fixed arrangements of cellular connections that exist in the brain.'' Hence, lobotomy. The problem with the theory was that it had no basis in fact. Moniz had just made it up, mixing together subjective observations of patients (he noted that many of them exhibited what he considered repetitious and stereotyped behavior) and his own interpretation of the work of others, including Pavlov, whom he cited in support of the theory. There was no hard evidence he could present to back up his ideas. He couldn't establish the existence of such fixed patterns of neurons and he certainly couldn't establish their role in the behavior of the mentally ill. Moniz's approach, ironically, defined a problem that was far more subtle than the solution. If there were such things as fixed patterns of neurons in the frontal lobes, causing particular kinds of behavior, they would have constituted an extremely specific kind of cerebral localization. A frontal lobotomy was clearly too crude a procedure for accurately interrupting such a remarkable configuration of cells. It would be like weeding a garden with a hand grenade.

The tragedy is that Moniz was not recognized and rejected as a charlatan for his psychosurgery work, the Franz Joseph Gall of the twentieth century. Not only was he not dismissed as a dangerous eccentric, he was embraced as a visionary. His ideas and his operation were taken up with enthusiasm, and in 1949 he was awarded the Nobel Prize in Medicine for his pioneering work in psychosurgery.

Moniz's appeal is not hard to understand. The lobotomy was a treatment aimed at patients who had been considered untreatable. The schizophrenics and other severely mentally ill persons originally deemed appropriate subjects for psychosurgery were chronic cases who filled half of all the hospital beds in the United States. For the patients, the lobotomy offered the possibility of relief from their disabling symptoms. For their families, it offered a possible end to the strain, and the hope that the patients might return to normal life. For the hospitals and mental institutions, it offered the chance to empty beds and, if not that, the possibility of bringing unruly patients under control. For the doctors, it was something they could actually do, a step they could take in the face of previously intractable disorders. It gave them power in an area where they had been powerless. At the beginning, then, the lobotomy appeared to be all things to all people, a genuine miracle cure that met the needs of both individuals and institutions.

Moniz directed only about one hundred lobotomies himself. His activity in the field was drastically curtailed when he was shot in the spine and crippled by a former patient. But his work inspired many others, most notably Walter Freeman and James W. Watts, a neurologist and a neurosurgeon at George Washington University in Washington, D.C., who emerged as the world's foremost practitioners and proponents of psychosurgery. Freeman and Watts performed their first operation, the first in the United States on September 14, 1936. By 1942, they had produced a textbook on the subject and by 1950, when they revised their book, they had performed more than one thousand operations.

"Psychosurgery has come of age," wrote Freeman and Watts in 1950, and their book, *Psychosurgery in the Treatment of Mental Disorders and Intractable Pain*, documents that belief in horrifying detail. Filled with case histories, photographs of patients, technical illustrations of operative techniques, X rays, charts, and graphs, the book presents psychosurgery as an evolved and evolving subspecialty of major medical and social importance. In a matter-of-fact tone full of confidence and optimism, the text deals with every aspect of lobotomy, from the selection of patients to the effect of the operation on the creative skills of painters, writers, and musicians. In the end, with some reservations, lobotomy emerges as a treatment for everything from "childhood schizophrenia" to unemployment. ("He worried because he couldn't find a job and he couldn't find a job because he worried so much. Lobotomy broke this vicious circle and he found both a job and peace of mind," reads the caption under a photograph of Case 76, a thirty-five-year-old lawyer operated on in 1940.) Obviously secure and sure of their place in the medical establishment, the authors only briefly acknowledge the growing criticism of psychosurgery, dismissing it as a form of apathy on the part of do-nothing types more interested in "symptomatologic minutiae" than in helping people.

Freeman and Watts's faith in psychosurgery was absolute. They made it the center of their careers and in the process they systematically abused their patients, the power they wielded as doctors, and even the existing knowledge of the brain and its functions. To take the least of the offenses first, Freeman and Watts, like Moniz before them, cited a variety of research studies done by others, many of which had nothing at all to do with psychosurgery and weren't intended to. In referring to these essentially benign observations in connection with their own work, Freeman and Watts were guilty of an insidious kind of exploitation bordering on deceit. Enlisting even the most fundamental works in neuroanatomy in the cause of psychosurgery was intellectually dishonest. Surely the neuroanatomists Constantin von Economo and G.N. Koskinas never meant for their brilliant maps of the cerebral cortex to serve as blueprints for the crude experiments of ambitious lobotomists. But that is exactly what they became in the hands of Freeman and Watts.

Over the years, Freeman and Watts developed criteria for identifying good candidates for lobotomy and listed various characteristics that they associated with improved chances for success. More women than men were able to leave institutions after surgery, they found, and they posited that this was because the women were afforded "greater protection" in the home. Older patients were good candidates provided they were not too demented, while children were "difficult to influence" and required the maximum operation. (Freeman and Watts had three grades of lobotomy that they performed—minimal, standard, and radical.) College-educated persons showed better results than those with only a grade school education, while those with high school education showed "many successes" and "some failures." The proportion of black females who benefited from the operation was greater than the proportion of white females. Jews showed the highest success rates, a fact the doctors attributed to "the greater family solidarity manifested by these people."

Besides schizophrenia, the diagnosis in the majority of Freeman and Watts's cases, the mental disorders for which lobotomy was an appropriate treatment, according to them, included involutional depression (prolonged, middle-age depression) and manic depression. "Best results may be expected in chronic anxiety states and obsessive tension states with or without compulsions," they wrote, "although disagreeable behavior may be expected as a result of unleashed hostility and may require a long period to subside." Freeman and Watts went on at length about the different kinds of affective disorders and types of schizophrenia, as they were understood in their time, and they emphasized the need for different operations in different cases. They also prescribed the lobotomy as a treatment for intractable pain caused by various organic diseases, noting that the pain persisted after psychosurgery but that the patient's relationship to the pain was changed. "Prefrontal lobotomy changes the attitude of the individual toward his pain," they wrote, "but does not alter the perception of pain. Whereas previous to operation it occupied the focus of his attention, after lobotomy pain fades into the background."

What all of this brings to mind, of course, is the fact that the criteria of which Freeman and Watts boast in 1950 came into existence only as the result of hundreds and hundreds of lobotomies performed on a trial-and-error basis. From the start, Freeman and Watts were experimenting, but they didn't let that slow their pace—within three months of their first operation they had already done twenty more lobotomies. What they did was make it all up as they went along, creating their specialty in the operating room. Their techniques, their criteria, their theories about the frontal lobes and the effect of lobotomy on the human mind and personality were all developed in a few frenetic years under a self-imposed pressure.

Freeman and Watts reported many failures in the early days as they sought the most efficient kind of operation. Again and again they devised new ways and places to cut the brains of their patients, only to be disappointed with the results. "We learned by experience that the incisions should not be made too far behind the coronal suture, at least in the upper quadrants," they wrote as they explained how cutting the brain too far back from the forehead left the patients inert, incontinent, and with "other indications of severe damage to the frontal lobes.'' (The coronal suture, which arcs across the top of the head from temple to temple, is the seam near the front of the skull where the bones join.) When they finally came up with a basic operation that satisfied them, they called it the ''precision method.''

In the standard lobotomy, Freeman and Watts made two burr holes, one on each side of the skull, just above the temples. After cutting through the dura and making a small incision in the cerebral cortex, they inserted into the brain an instrument called a leucotome, which was much like a thin table knife with a rounded end. They then made what they called ''sweeping cuts'' with the leukotome, slicing through the white matter in the upper and the lower portions of the frontal lobes. After the sweeping cuts they removed the thin leukotome and, using a wider and blunter knife, made stablike cuts that extended the sweeping cuts deeper into the brain. The procedure was carried out on both sides of the brain. The radical lobotomy was the same, except the approach was made slightly farther back from the front of the brain. In the minimal operation the sweeping cuts in the upper parts of the frontal lobes were eliminated. So, while the gray matter of a lobotomized brain would have just two small incisions on each side, the underlying white matter would be virtually sliced in two, the front of it cut off from the rest.

On occasion, Freeman and Watts operated while their patients were under local anesthesia. That is, they performed prefrontal lobotomies on severely mentally ill patients while those patients were awake. They did it, they said, to monitor the progressive effects of the various cuts as the operation proceeded and the immediate effect of the operation as a whole. The patient's level of ''disorientation'' was an intraoperative indicator they used in some cases to determine whether sufficient tissue had been cut. During the surgery they would engage in extensive conversations with the patients. Periodically they would put them through standard routines to test their degree of orientation—counting down from one hundred by sevens, singing ''God Bless America,'' naming makes

of automobiles, and so on. They also discussed what was
happening during the operation and questioned the patients about their condition and their state of mind. While
brain surgery under local anesthesia was not uncommon,
it was usually carried out on mentally healthy patients as
a way of studying cerebral localization. As the surgeons
stimulated the cortex with electrodes, the patients would
report the effects—twitching fingers or toes, the arousal
of a specific memory or mental image. The conversations
recorded by Freeman and Watts were something else altogether. Transcripts reveal them as eerie exchanges with an
oddly casual tone. Punctuated by the patients' sometimes
surreal, sometimes poetic, always disturbing comments,
they provide a stark glimpse into a truly strange place.

The following conversation took place during a ''standard'' lobotomy performed on a thirty-six-year-old man
in the summer of 1943. Diagnosed a schizophrenic, the
man had been ill for about a year, according to the case
history. His illness had been marked by a suicide attempt, long hours spent ''thinking about the devil,'' the
belief that he had syphilis, and the belief that the FBI
was following him.

The patient was under good control and had been
talking freely, relevantly, and coherently concerning
his emotional difficulties. When asked if he was afraid
that he would do something terrible he replied: ''Yes,
there is a fear there. It is not a desire. I might do
something wrong and not know it was wrong. It didn't
seem possible that I'd make fifty decisions all of them
wrong. It seemed to be caused by self-centeredness,
thinking of myself instead of others. I haven't done the
right thing in not helping others.''

DOCTOR: If you weren't worried, do you think you
could help others?

PATIENT: It would be better to help others than to
think of the bad things I've done.

(The openings were completed, and the patient was
quiet, blood pressure 106/70, pulse 72. Sweeping incisions were made on the left side, in the upper and
lower quadrants.)

DOCTOR: Do you feel any difference?

PATIENT: I feel there's a book on my face. They worked on the left side. There was a drawing when they put the knife in.

DOCTOR: Did you feel it on the right side?

PATIENT: No.

DOCTOR: Did you feel it behind the eye?

PATIENT: No.

(Sweeping incisions were made in the right upper and lower quadrants. The patient was able to respond promptly, blood pressure 98/70, pulse 76; he was not nauseated.)

DOCTOR: How do you feel?

PATIENT: Not too bad, Doc. I feel like I was slit in two. Well I'd rather open my eyes, and only the left one is open. Is that Mr. Wilkinson?

DOCTOR: How does that feel?

PATIENT: That's all right. (He is still approximately oriented.)

DOCTOR: How about that feeling in your head?

PATIENT: That seems to be gone.

DOCTOR: When did it go?

PATIENT: A few minutes ago.

DOCTOR: What happened to it?

PATIENT: I don't know, Doc. It just disappeared.

DOCTOR: Are your worries gone?

PATIENT: My worries? What worries? I know what you mean. I guess they are.

DOCTOR: Why did you let yourself worry?

PATIENT: I don't know, Doc. There wasn't ever a time I wanted to.

DOCTOR: Couldn't you do something about it?

PATIENT: I was never able to do so before, Doc.

DOCTOR: You wasted a lot of time, didn't you?

PATIENT: No, I spent a lot of time over in the hospital trying to get well.

(Stab incisions were made on the right side of the quadrants. Patient voided on the table while the lower incisions were being made.)

DOCTOR: When did you go to the hospital?

PATIENT: June 1942, three months then, and three months after July 1943, when I came home.

DOCTOR: Did you receive shock treatments?

PATIENT: No, no treatment at all.

DOCTOR: Did you think it was a waste of time?

PATIENT: I think that's their method. I don't think they neglect you. The doctor would come through every day and glance at you and ask a few questions, but that was all.

(Radial stabs were completed on left side.)

PATIENT: Something snapped just then. I'll wait until he's satisfied. Can you put that stuff in my head?

DOCTOR: They're washing out now. Do you feel anything in your head?

PATIENT: No.

DOCTOR: Does your head feel empty?

PATIENT: No, I didn't feel anything just then.

DOCTOR: What day is this?

PATIENT: Friday, August the something or other. (Stirring a little bit uneasily.)

DOCTOR: What is 100 minus 7:

PATIENT: 93, 86, 79, 72, 65, 58, 51, 44, 37, 30, 23, 16, 9, 2. (Rapidly and correctly.)

DOCTOR: Name all the autos you can in one minute.

(Patient names eight in thirty seconds and none later. He is quieter, less responsive; voice has changed in the past few moments.)

DOCTOR: What is happening now?

PATIENT: Don't they believe in this stuff? God, that hurts!

DOCTOR: What's going on?

PATIENT: I'm being operated on. Doctor Watts, isn't it?

DOCTOR: Any comments?

PATIENT: Only that it hurts. Nothing much to do about it.

DOCTOR: They're sewing up. Are you glad it's over?

PATIENT: Uh-huh. That's the end of it—whew!

DOCTOR: Does your conscience hurt?

PATIENT: I don't know where it is. It was down by my heart, but I can't feel it at all.

DOCTOR: Do you notice any change due to the operation?

PATIENT: I don't know yet. I'm still flat on my back. It does seem to stop that pain on the right side of my head. I was getting thoughts from my mother.

DOCTOR: What thoughts?

PATIENT: I can't remember now. All I can say is they were working through my head.

DOCTOR: Did your mother know best?

PATIENT: Not particularly. I feel it is part of the necessity of the time. Up until a couple of days ago my heart beat backwards to everybody but her. Now I can't feel my heart at all. Put my hands over there soon.

DOCTOR: Are you glad you were operated?

PATIENT: I think so. Yes, sir.

DOCTOR: Why?

PATIENT: Because I've got a chance now. Before I didn't have any.

At 11 A.M. the sutures are in and the drapes taken off; the patient is relaxed and smiling.

Three days after the operation the patient was back to his old self. He was inert, and when the doctors managed to bring him out of it he spoke only of his delusions. "He says that the peculiar sensation in his head is gone and that the Devil is not with him," the report reads, "but nevertheless he is not able to talk in any coherent manner at the present time, although he is thoroughly oriented." Freeman and Watts concluded that "the nucleus of schizophrenic ideas with this particular emotional set had evidently spread over a larger area and that the fantasy activities were unchecked." They decided that relief for a "confirmed schizophrenic" required a more radical lobotomy "so that practically the whole imaginative life of the individual has to be sacrificed in order to get rid of the pathologic fantasy." They theorized that in the early stages of schizophrenia, or in an "acute process," the standard operation might be sufficient but that "the prerequisite for success in this case is destruction of the fantasy life." They hadn't cut enough, and five days after the first operation they performed another, more radical lobotomy. And, again, the patient was awake the whole time.

Reoperation was undertaken . . . approximately 1.5 cm. behind the original incisions. During the early parts of the procedure he was somewhat retarded and afraid of the same obsessive thoughts that he had had previously.

DOCTOR: Did you think yourself contaminated?

PATIENT: Yes.

DOCTOR: What did the experts say about it?

PATIENT: They didn't tell me. They might have told my mother or my brother.

DOCTOR: You didn't believe your mother or your brother?

PATIENT: No, I wanted to, but I couldn't. It didn't work.

DOCTOR: So, in addition to being a rotter, you were diseased and a doubter?

PATIENT: Yes.

DOCTOR: Everything.

PATIENT: I had 'em all.

DOCTOR: You wanted to kill yourself?

PATIENT: Yes, I thought that was what they wanted me to do, and I didn't see anything else to do.

DOCTOR: Then you added up to a coward and a failure?

PATIENT: It seems that way, Doctor.

DOCTOR: And then became quietly insane.

PATIENT: Doctor, that's putting it mildly.

DOCTOR: Are you facing death now?

PATIENT: Yes.

DOCTOR: Anything else?

PATIENT: No, I trust you. I know you're doing the best you can for me.

(The left medial and lateral cuts were made. The patient was quiet and relaxed. Pulse 66. Blood pressure 108/70. He was somewhat nauseated. Correctly oriented.)

DOCTOR: Lloyd?

PATIENT: Huh?

DOCTOR: How do you feel now?

PATIENT: It's like a tingling in the top of my head now.

DOCTOR: Is it like the Devil?

PATIENT: Uh-huh.

DOCTOR: Does it go down to your toes?

PATIENT: Yes.

DOCTOR: Which side?

PATIENT: Both sides.

DOCTOR: Is it your privates?

PATIENT: Yes, Doctor.

DOCTOR: What's that like?

PATIENT: Feels like the devil.

DOCTOR: Do you feel the devil castrating you?

PATIENT: Yes.

DOCTOR: Or just masturbating you?

PATIENT: Just masturbating, I guess.

(Stabs are made on the right side. He retches and tries to vomit without success. His voice becomes toneless, and it is difficult to get him to respond.)

DOCTOR: Who's talking to you?

PATIENT: Doctor Freeman.

DOCTOR: Have you been operated on?

PATIENT: Yes.

DOCTOR: What operation?

No answer.

DOCTOR: What's being done to you?

PATIENT: Huh? Oh, they're working on my head.

DOCTOR: Why?

PATIENT: To see what's wrong with it.

DOCTOR: What's wrong?

PATIENT: I don't know, Doc.

DOCTOR: Anything serious?

PATIENT: Yes.

DOCTOR: What's wrong?

No answer.

DOCTOR: Are devils in it?

PATIENT: Yeah. He could probably be as much with a couple of wits in the right place as another person could with a couple of weeks of training.

DOCTOR: Are you full of corruption?
PATIENT: Uh-huh.
DOCTOR: Do you want to kill yourself?
PATIENT: Yeah.
DOCTOR: Does the devil tell you to get well?
PATIENT: Yeah.
DOCTOR: Why does he do this?
PATIENT: So he'd be boss.
DOCTOR: Subtract 7 from 100 down the line.
PATIENT: 93, 84, 73, 62, 51, 50, 42, 41, 50 (pauses), 50, 50, 50, 50, 50, 50, 42, 42, 41, 40, 32, 31, 30, 22, 21, 20, 18, 19, 20, 2, 1, 0. (His voice is flat, his replies brief.)
DOCTOR: What's my name?
PATIENT: Stewart.
DOCTOR: What hospital is this?
PATIENT: I don't know.
DOCTOR: What day is this?
PATIENT: Thursday. (Incorrect).
DOCTOR: Were you operated on?
PATIENT: No.

Upon recovering from the operation and returning home the patient was described as indolent and sarcastic. He was incontinent and gained forty pounds. He returned to his job as a draftsman but was fired within two years for inefficiency. Four years after the surgery his brother, with whom he was living, reported that he had lost all sense of time, spent four to six hours a day washing his hands, wore dirty clothes, ate sloppily, and resented being corrected. He also drank too much and talked constantly. Freeman and Watts concluded that they had in fact succeeded in freeing the patient from his obsessions, delusions, and "a whole welter of psychotic abnormalities." They described him as "an intelligent, extroverted individual in perfect harmony with himself and utterly useless to his family." They were pleased to note that his aggressive misbehavior was limited to drinking, which they attributed to his lack of imagination. In the end, Freeman and Watts were chiefly interested in this case because of the conversations carried on

during the two procedures. "The difference in the alert-
ness, coherence and cogency of his replies may serve to
explain some of the functions of this narrow slab of tissue
lying between the two incisions," they wrote.

In their presentation and analysis of these cases, Freeman and Watts seem oblivious to the extreme circumstances they are describing and the bizarre nature of the
conversations. Asking a patient if he felt the devil masturbating him during his second lobotomy in five days
was apparently routine for them. So routine, in fact, that
they then attempted to measure and compare the coherence and cogency of the replies to such questions. In the
final conversation included here, Freeman and Watts
added sound effects to the transcript. They did this, they
explained in their book, "to indicate the abrupt change
from panicky apprehension to calm indifference following incision of the third quadrant (left lower), and disorientation following the radial stab incisions into the
final quadrant (right lower)." The patient was a twenty-
four-year-old man diagnosed as a schizophrenic.

9:30 A.M. Towel sutures going in. Frank is quiet
except for grunting and groaning. He was alert and
smiling earlier, but now is tense and overventilating;
his hands are cold and clammy. Pulse: 68; Blood Pressure: 102/56. He repeats over and over: "O I'm goin',
I'm goin, I can't breathe."

DOCTOR: Are your (sic) scared?

PATIENT: Yeh.

DOCTOR: What of?

PATIENT: I don't know, Doctor.

DOCTOR: What do you want?

PATIENT: Not a lot. I just want friends. That's all.
How long's this going on?

DOCTOR: Two hours.

PATIENT: Two hours? I can't last that long. (Squeezes
hand.)

DOCTOR: How do you feel?

PATIENT: I don't feel anything but they're cutting me
now.

DOCTOR: You wanted it?

PATIENT: Yes, but I didn't think you'd do it awake. O gee whiz, I'm dying. O doctor. Please stop. O God. I'm goin again. Oh, oh, oh. Ow. (Chisel) Oh, this is awful. Ow. (He grabs my hand and sinks his nails into it.) O, God, I'm goin, please stop.

DOCTOR: Frank?

PATIENT: Yeh?

DOCTOR: What work have you done?

PATIENT: O, a little bit of everything.

DOCTOR: Such as what?

PATIENT: Brakeman on a railroad. That was a good job. Ow . . . and a material checker . . . ow . . . stop, unh, unh, unh. I liked that one, too. Hey listen, cut it out for God's sake. O, quit. I'm goin. What's goin on . . . Hey, give me some air (The towels have slipped a bit). Hey, what's goin on? O, please stop.

DOCTOR: Relax!

PATIENT: I can't relax. Oh, what's goin on here? (Rongeur.) (Admits he feels no pain.) Hey this is . . . O, you know I can't go on. O, I'm having trouble breathing. O, stop experimenting.

DOCTOR: Stop what?

PATIENT: I don't know. How long's this been goin on? Fix it up. I'm having trouble breathing.

(Blood pressure 136/44. Pulse 76)

DOCTOR: Feel better now?

PATIENT: No, I'm getting worse. I'm goin. O, come on, will you?

DOCTOR: How much is 100 (minus) 7?

PATIENT: 93, unh, unh. Ow! (Tapping) 86—79—72—65—. (Drilling) Ow! I don't know. Give me some air, air, air. Ow! Hey, cut it out. Cut it out! (Trembling hands still cold. He is quick to grab my hand when I try to take it away.)

DOCTOR: How do you feel?

PATIENT: Yes, sir. Click.

DOCTOR: What's it like?

PATIENT: Oh, a pickle, puffle phl, (sic) hey stop it will ya?

DOCTOR: You're grabbing me awful tight.

PATIENT: Am I? I can't help it. How long does this go on? (Right lower cuts)

DOCTOR: Glad you're being operated?

PATIENT: Yes, it makes me feel better.

DOCTOR: Why the fuss?

PATIENT: Oh, I can't help it. I can't breathe. Hey, what are you doing there?

(Right upper cuts)

DOCTOR: Feel all right now?

PATIENT: Yeah, I can't breathe. Hey, when is this thing over?

DOCTOR: What will you do when you're well?

PATIENT: O, go back to work. Oh, I can't stand it.

DOCTOR: What job?

PATIENT: O, it's a good job, brakeman with a railroad.

DOCTOR: Scared?

PATIENT: Yeh.

DOCTOR: Sing God Bless America.

PATIENT: (He starts rather high and does a couple of lines, then grunts and continues with his chatter.) Ow! That's hot. What's going on here? (Warm saline.)

(Left lower cut)

(Left upper cut)

(Stabs left)

DOCTOR: Was that hot?

PATIENT: No, it wasn't hot.

DOCTOR: How do you feel?

PATIENT: Yes, yes.

10:15 A.M. He is moving his head about during the stabs, especially when the knife touches the dura.

(Stabs right) (Voice suddenly becomes muffled.)

DOCTOR: Who's operating?

PATIENT: I dunno.

DOCTOR: Are you comfortable?

PATIENT: No.

DOCTOR: Why do you jerk around?

PATIENT: I don't know.

DOCTOR: Can you breathe?

PATIENT: Yes. (He thumps with his hands which are now quite warm and pink.)

DOCTOR: Feel fine?
PATIENT: Yeh, pretty good.
DOCTOR: What's my name?
PATIENT: Doctor John Silvia Silberg.
DOCTOR: Wrong. What's my name?
PATIENT: Dr. John Silvia.
DOCTOR: What place is this?
PATIENT: George Washington Hospital.
DOCTOR: What are you doing here?
PATIENT: Being operated on.
DOCTOR: What for?
PATIENT: There's something wrong with the brain. I don't know what it is.
DOCTOR: Is it all right now?
PATIENT: Where's the door?
DOCTOR: Afraid?
PATIENT: No.
DOCTOR: What's happened to your fear?
PATIENT: Gone.
DOCTOR: Why were you afraid?
PATIENT: I don't know.
DOCTOR: Feel okay?
PATIENT: Yes. I feel pretty good now.

As bad as the operations under local anesthesia were, the most outrageous single development in the whole outrageous psychosurgery era was the transorbital lobotomy, as refined and implemented by the neurologist Walter Freeman. The transorbital lobotomy was a gruesome surgical technique in which an instrument identical to an ice pick was passed in over the eyeball and poked through the back of the eye socket (technically known as the orbit) and into the frontal lobes. The ice pick was then twisted back and forth and up and down to destroy brain tissue. The procedure was carried out on both the left and the right side of the brain. In a weird, wholly inappropriate application of the kind of good old American know-how that gave us the automobile assembly line, Freeman developed the transorbital lobotomy to the point where he was able to perform as many as twenty-five operations in a single day. He described his method as "simple, quick, effective, and safe to be entrusted to the psychiatrist." What Freeman did was reduce the lobotomy to a routine, minor procedure that could be performed by nonsurgeons. His associate Watts, the neurosurgeon, split with him on this, holding that any procedure involving the cutting of brain tissue was major surgery and should be left to the specialist.

In practice, Freeman's "quick" brain surgery was as terrible as it sounds. He used three electroshocks, both to knock the patient out and because he believed that the shocks also disorganized the "cortical patterns" that were supposedly the underlying cause of the patient's problem. Once the patient was unconscious, Freeman merely lifted the eyelid and stuck in the ice pick, bedding it against the bone at the back of the socket. (For his first few transorbitals, Freeman used an actual ice pick—"this humble instrument," he called it. Later, a surgical version was developed, with the shaft marked off in centimeters to show the depth of penetration into the brain.) After placing the ice pick at the correct angle—an angle he determined by eye—Freeman tapped it through the bone and into the brain with a small hammer. He then made the "cuts."

Freeman's writings on the transorbital lobotomy are rife with technical details and measurements that imply a degree of precision that was plainly nonexistent. As an example, here is Freeman's *complete* description of his technique.

When the patient is unconscious I pinch the upper eyelid between thumb and finger and bring it well away from the eyeball. I then insert the point of the transorbital leucotome into the conjunctival sac, taking care not to touch the skin or lashes, and move the point around until it settles against the vault of the orbit. I then drop to one knee, beside the table, in order to aim the instrument parallel with the bony ridge of the nose, and slightly toward the midline. When the 5 cm. mark is reached, I pull the handle of the instrument as far laterally as the rim of the orbit will permit in order to sever fibers at the base of the frontal lobe. I then return the instrument half way to its previous position and drive it further to a depth of 7 cm. from the margin of the upper eyelid. Again I sight the instrument as carefully as possible, and take a profile photograph of it in this position. This is the nearest approach to precision of which the method can boast. Then comes the ticklish part. Arteries are within reach. Keeping the instrument in the frontal plane, I move it 15° to 20° medially and about 30° laterally, return it to the mid position, and withdraw by a twisting movement, at the same time exercising considerable pressure on the eyelids to prevent hemorrhage. I then proceed with the opposite side, using an identical instrument, but freshly sterilized, because some germs might be carried away from the lashes or skin of the first side operated upon.

Freeman's description makes it sound like a lot more is going on than the scrambling of human brains with an ice pick, but that is exactly all there was to it. And, like Moniz's theory of "fixed neuronal patterns," there is something essentially off about Freeman's whole concept of the transorbital lobotomy. How could it possibly be important to perform psychosurgery "quickly"? Unless of course the priority was to clear out overcrowded institutions without resorting to the services of neurosurgeons. Critics of psychosurgery have charged over the years that emptying the mental hospitals was in fact the main reason the lobotomy became so widespread. Freeman and Watts were particularly conscious of the situation in the large mental institutions, and several times in their work they refer to the positive impact psychosurgery could have on these institutions. "As we have stated previously . . . the problem of the disturbed ward of the state hospital can be all but solved by the performance of prefrontal lobotomy on a large scale," they wrote. They promoted the transorbital lobotomy in particular as a technique ideally suited for use in crowded mental hospitals, "where it is obviously of greatest value." Indeed, when Freeman and Watts were analyzing their results, their chief measure of success was whether or not the patient was able to leave the institution.

Analysis of results was another controversial area. Writing in the 1985 edition of their book *Behavioral Neu-*

rology, Drs. Jonathan H. Pincus and Gary J. Tucker point out some basic problems with the medical literature dealing with psychosurgery. "It is surprising that, despite the large number of patients who underwent frontal lobotomy in the 1940s and 1950s before effective drugs were available, very little was learned about the efficacy of the procedure. Several basic medical questions have never been satisfactorily answered: What were the indications for the procedure? What were the complications and what was their incidence? What changes in the patients could be measured by pre- and post-operative psychological evaluation? What were the long-term results? One of the critical deficiencies has been the lack of a truly controlled study." Pincus and Tucker then nail down the fundamental flaw. "In many instances," they note, "the selection of patients for frontal lobotomy, the operation and the post-operative evaluation were performed by the same individuals."

Naturally, Freeman and Watts evaluated their own results, a stunning exercise in subjective analysis. The main chart in their book looks like this:

RESULTS OF PREFRONTAL LOBOTOMY—1949

DIAGNOSIS	NUMBER	GOOD	FAIR	POOR	DEATHS	
					OPERATIVE	LATER*
		%	%	%	%	
Schizophrenias	328	35	38	25	2	8
Involutional Psychoses	147	60	24	14	2	20
Obsessive and Psycho- neuroses	121	57	28	11	4	5
Pain cases	21	43	38		19	7
Total	617	45	33	19	3	40

*Later deaths are not included in the tabulations.
All patients were traced in 1949-50.

Freeman and Watts never spell out exactly what they mean by Good, Fair, and Poor. They simply state that each case was judged on its own merits, and that a result judged Good in one set of circumstances might be only Fair, given another set of circumstances. Variables that played a role in their decisions included the diagnosis, the patient's family situation, the course and duration of the illness, and the period of institutionalization. What is most glaringly obvious is the inadequacy of the classification system—Good, Fair, and Poor define a range too simple and too vague for even a grammar school marking system, never mind a system for measuring the degress of success of psychosurgery. And such vagueness permeates Freeman and Watt's analysis of their results. Nevertheless, upon evaluating 617 cases they confidently concluded that "Five out of six patients, including both sexes, all ages, and all diagnoses, are considered as improved by prefrontal lobotomy." The chart above was provided in support of that remarkable conclusion.

Even though Freeman and Watts put the best possible face on their results, they managed to get only 45 percent of their cases into the Good category. By their own admission, they wound up with less than optimum results more than half the time. And in a section on failures they state that one hundred of their first five hundred cases, or 20 percent, had to be considered failures. That they considered such figures acceptable, and even something to be proud of, illustrates just how comfortable the psychosurgeons were in the world.

They were comfortable enough to think nothing of performing a lobotomy on a four-year-old boy and then listing him as "improved" in spite of the fact that he died of meningitis three weeks after the operation. (In their account of the case, Freeman and Watts coldly note that "Necropsy showed clean healing wounds," a bald attempt to escape blame for the death.) They were comfortable enough to perform two lobotomies on a six-year-old girl in the space of seven months and three lobotomies on a seventeen-year-old in a year. Though the girl was found to be almost completely withdrawn from her environment four years after surgery, the doctors considered her "improved" because she was "less troublesome" as a lobotomized ten-year-old than she had been as a disturbed six-year-old. "In spite of her increased speed and strength," they wrote, "she can be more easily managed at home, is beginning to put sentences together and the impulsive, destructive behavior is subsiding." The seventeen-year-old remained in a state hospital, one of their admitted failures.

It was the advent of antipsychotic drugs in the 1950s that brought an end to the age of psychosurgery. But what endures from that time, as UCLA's Arnold Scheibel has pointed out, is a relative ignorance about the nature of mental illness and its treatments. More than thirty years after their introduction, antipsychotic drugs remain the primary treatment for schizophrenia, and they are still notably crude when measured against the complexity of the brain's chemistry. No one who prescribes the drugs knows exactly how or why they work, or even if they will work in any given case. The drugs are easily misused—either overprescribed or inappropriately prescribed—and some critics consider them nothing more than a "chemical straightjacket." "It is generally recognized that there are too many antipsychotic drugs available, and that this makes rational prescribing difficult," wrote the authors of *A Handbook of Psychoactive Medicines*, a 1982 British publication. And in the *Schizophrenia Bulletin* in 1987, Dr. John M. Kane noted that "Despite the introduction of a variety of different antipsychotics and chemical classes of antipsychotics over the past 30 years, there are at present no convincing data that among medications currently marketed in the United States any one is more effective either in schizophrenia in general or in specific subtypes of the disorder."

"Each of the major so-called tranquilizers, thorazine and the others, has its own slightly different signatures," Scheibel has said. "Some will work on one patient, some will work on another. And nobody has the faintest notion. And when I say work, what they do is make life more liveable. They're not treatments, right? They're palliatives." So, we are beyond the ice pick, but we are just beyond it. Though antipsychotic drugs control some of schizophrenia's symptoms in some cases, they are blunt, inexact instruments. In spite of what they can do for the patients, it's what they can't do for them that is most obvious—they can't cure them or give them back the lives they might have had.

Not surprisingly, schizophrenia is a research-intensive specialty. One way to grasp the range of projects underway is to use the computer analogy. Some of the work involves hardware, the anatomy and biochemistry of the brain; some of it involves software, the nature and structure of thought and the stages of the thinking process. Spurred on by the new technologies, the borders between the two area are blurring, and it is in the inevitable merger of biology and psychology that hope for a more complete understanding of schizophrenia lies.

Scheibel and a UCLA colleague, Joyce Kovelman, made an important contribution on the hardware side when they discovered badly disorganized cells in the hippocampi of a group of schizophrenic brains they were studying. Today, Scheibel and his team are pursuing this "structural anomaly." They know when in the course of embryonic development it is likely to occur, and now they are trying to establish how it happens. They suspect that viruses, simple flu viruses and others, that strike mothers with weakened immunities early in the second trimester of pregnancy are involved. "Perhaps," Scheibel notes, "maternal exposure to or infection by a common virus in this critical window period may be responsible for a very significant number—who knows, maybe all—of the youngsters who later became schizophrenic."

Even as they work on their own particular piece of the puzzle, researchers like Scheibel are never far removed from the larger reality of schizophrenia. The disease has many dimensions, encompassing everything from microbiology to sociology, from the workings of a single gene to the problems of homeless psychotics. And the elements can never be completely separated from each other. One sad detail reinforces this: of the ten brains Scheibel examined in his original study, three were the brains of suicides.

The best-known and most firmly established fact about the physiologic substrata of schizophrenia is that the brains of schizophrenics show excessive dopamine activity. Dopamine is the neurotransmitter that has also been linked to Parkinson's disease, but in the case of Parkinson's, it's a shortage of dopamine activity that is the problem. The dopamine connection in schizophrenia was made when it was noted that patients taking antipsychotic drugs tended to develop the tremors and shaking that are characteristic of Parkinson's disease as their schizophrenia symptoms abated. Not enough dopamine meant Parkinson's, too much dopamine meant schizophrenia. The assumption was that the antipsychotic drugs were blocking the uptake of dopamine by the brain, which eased the schizophrenia symptoms but brought on the Parkinson's symptoms. Research established that this was indeed the case. Exactly how excessive dopamine activity contributes to the thought disorders that are seen in schizophrenia is not known, and as Keith Nuechterlein, another UCLA schizophrenia researcher, points out, the brain's complexity does not allow for simple conclusions. While it is suspected that there may be as many as two hundred neurotransmitters active in the brain, only some thirty of them have been identified. "Tracking backwards from successful treatments is always hazardous," Nuechterlein has said. "You know that if a treatment is successful you've affected some link in the causal chain, but which link? Are you way down the path from the original etiology, or are you close? It's tough."

As the director of the Aftercare Clinic of the UCLA Neuropsychiatric Institute, Nuechterlein is involved in both the ongoing clinical care of schizophrenics and in research into the nature and causes of the disease. He has been working in the field for fifteen years as a psychologist, and he has been in a position to observe the merging of disciplines that marks current schizophrenia research. "What you're talking about is studying the metabolic underpinning of mental activity," explained Nuechterlein. "And so the question 'Is something a psychological phenomenon or is it a physiological phenomenon?' is becoming, more and more, not a terribly meaningful question. For those cases of schizophrenia that have a genetic component, which is probably most cases, there is an ultimate component that is clearly biological. As the genes release their first biochemical products, those aren't thoughts. But schizophrenia is a disorder of thinking and feeling, so it is classifiable at that level.''

Nuechterlein's expertise is in the structure of thought and thought processes, and much of the research he is involved in concerns the role of attention in schizophrenia. Technically, the term *attention* refers to much more than the ability to stay awake during a boring lecture, though that is certainly part of it. Attention is a critical component in all forms of thinking, or, as psychologists refer to it, cognitive processing. Nuechterlein's work posits a ''fundamental disturbance of various aspects of attention'' as the critical factor in some schizophrenic thought disorders. To explain that idea, Nuechterlein first distinguished between two different kinds of cognitive processing—the kind that requires effort and purpose and the kind that is automatic. He used speaking as an example of effortful cognitive processing. ''One thing that we're all doing when we are speaking,'' he said, ''is tracking what we just said. We know what our end point is and as we speak we keep assessing—'Is this going to bring me to the end of my sentence in a meaningful way? Is this sentence going to further the point I'm trying to make?' and so on.'' Such tracking is a part of many kinds of thinking, and though it might sound like something we do automatically, technically it requires conscious attention. Nuechterlein used driving as an example of the kind of ''overlearned'' things people do without paying conscious attention. ''If you're a practiced driver,'' he said, ''you can carry on a converation while you're driving and have it not be interrupted virtually at all unless something unexpected happens. Then you have to pull away part of your attentional capacity from the conversation and refocus that on your driving. And you stop talking. It's a very natural thing. You automatically stop talking because you can't do both at one time.'' In schizophrenia, Nuechterlein said, there might be problems either generating the initial attention required for effortful cognitive processing or maintaining that attention over the course of a task. If so, schizophrenics would not be capable of successfully "tracking" their thought processes. Such a disturbance might account for the "loose associations" that can characterize schizophrenic thinking and speech.

Another possibility Nuechterlein presented concerned a disturbance of "automatic" cognitive processing. It might be that schizophrenics are capable of effortful cognitive processing, but because of a problem with automatic cognitive processing, they are forced to pay attention to things that the rest of us don't have to and are overwhelmed by it all. "Think of the person who knows how to drive very well and can talk at the same time," Nuechterlein said. "All of a sudden, something happens and their driving skills get really poor. Now they have to be real careful and they can't talk and drive at the same time anymore. What if, during the process of moving towards schizophrenia, something happened with the brain and as a result things that were well learned, things you didn't have to devote any conscious attention to, all of a sudden those things did not happen automatically anymore. You would then have to devote more of your conscious processing to that and you wouldn't have as much left to do other things, like tracking."

Disturbances of attention do not account for all the symptoms of schizophrenia. Nuechterlein explained how another intriguing psychological phenomenon might be involved in some of schizophrenia's more florid symptoms, such as auditory hallucinations, thought insertions, and delusions, which are considered key components of the disease. "One way to pull some of these things together," he said, "Is that they involve a disturbance in the boundary between you and not you. The disturbance seems to be that things are penetrating into the boundary that is you, whereas you could usually control that."

Nuechterlein and his fellow schizophrenia researchers around the country and the world today are doing more than theorizing about the subtleties of thought structure and personality. They are using advanced brain imaging techniques and other technologies, like the EEG, to actually link the psychological manifestations of the disease with underlying anatomy and biochemistry. Because attention is known to be, at least in part, a function of the frontal lobes, researchers are trying to determine if lowered metabolic activity in the frontal lobes is a factor in schizophrenia. Their primary tool for this work is the PET scanner, today's most sophisticated brain imaging tool.

The schizophrenics who get PET scanned at the University of California at Irvine, where Nuechterlein sends his patients for the procedure, begin their long sessions by having electrodes stuck all over their heads and an IV line run into each arm. This prep work is done as they sit in a crowded corner of the crowded maze of offices, labs, and hallways that makes up the Brain Imaging Center there. If it is their first time, they must also be fitted with white plastic masks that are warmed and applied while soft so that they can be molded to their faces for a perfect fit. The masks, which look similar to the kind worn by hockey goalies, attach to the scanner and keep the patients' heads still while they are being scanned. Once they are prepped, with tubes and wires dangling, a rolling IV pole at their side, the patients carefully make their way over to the small store room that has been converted, by the placement of a piece of cardboard over a window, into the "uptake room." It is in the uptake room that the next step in the procedure takes place.

Unlike X-ray machines and CAT scanners, which beam things at the subject, PET scanners are passive and merely receive what is emanating from the subject. While X rays and CAT scans reveal structure, PET scans reveal function. PET stands for "positron emission tomography," and PET scanners work by detecting radiation emitted by decaying isotopes—positrons—that have been "taken up" by the subject's brain. In the uptake room at Irvine, the schizophrenic patient sits in an old, green easy chair. A jury-rigged black curtain isolates him from two technicians who draw blood from his left arm every fifteen seconds for the first three minutes that the isotope is dripping into him through the IV line in his right arm.

To keep track of the ever-decreasing amount of isotope in the blood, a total of twenty-four blood samples is taken over the course of the procedure. The electrodes on the patient's head are wired into an evoked potentials machine in the next room, which measures his brain's electrical activity. With the lights out, the patient sits and watches a screen as a series of blurred, single-digit numbers are flashed at him. His task is to push a button each time he sees a zero. The task, designed to test his attention capacity, goes on for half an hour. As he sits there, his brain mistakes the radioactive isotope for glucose and takes it up to burn for energy.

When the task is finished, the electrodes and the IV line in his right arm are removed, and the patient walks back down the hall to the scanning room. The remaining line in his left arm will be used for drawing more blood during the scan. The PET scanner is a large, square machine about shoulder height with a hole in the middle and a long table protruding from the front of it. The patient lies on the table and his mask is fitted over his face and notched into place on the table. Technicians then adjust the table, which will automatically inch the patient into the machine as the scanning proceeds. Starting at the crown of the head and working down, the scanner takes pictures of slices of the brain. The number of slices varies, usually they shoot about nine. What the PET scanner produces is a full-spectrum color portrait of the metabolic activity of the brain as it was during the uptake of the isotope. Even though the scanning is done after the numbers task is finished and takes nearly an hour, the pictures it generates reveal the brain's pattern of activity as it was while the schizophrenic patient was performing his task.

As the patient lies quietly in the machine, the work of the lab continues around him. Technicians monitor the scan, patients are prepped, doctors and staff pass in and out of the room. Scattered about on every available surface, dozens of the eerie white masks stare blankly out of the clutter of the proceedings. The names of the patients they fit are scribbled on them in pencil. Because the schizophrenics are often off their medications for the sake of the research studies, some of them hallucinate while they are being scanned. Others doze. Standing before the video monitor connected to the PET scanner, a doctor watches the pictures of the brain come up, one after the other, slice after slice. He speaks with excitement of all the scans they have been doing and all the ones they will be doing. He is inspired by the accumulation of this great mass of raw information. These brains will always be on file, and as the doctors and researchers learn more and more, they can go back and see what was there, look again and see what they didn't see the first time, or the tenth. The schizophrenic patient is lying there, his frontal lobes under scrutiny in a strange, modern echo of the lobotomy. The doctor is looking at that troubled brain, watching it work, seeing it think. It's quite a view, right there in front of him. As much as he sees, though, there's much more that he can't see. And he knows it.

CONCLUSION

As I think about the future of neurological medicine, it strikes me that twice in the course of researching this book I was bewitched. The first time it happened I began to see the world as a neurosurgeon sees it. The second time, I began to see the nervous system as a neuroscientist sees it. Both times, my reverie was broken by a contrary impulse, born of my civilian status, to think like a patient. I relate these experiences to the future of neurological medicine because they show how attitudes are formed, and it's the formation of attitudes, as much as anything, that defines the future.

I liked the way the best surgeons ran things during an operation. I admired and was impressed by the way they accepted responsibility for another human life. I liked their brand of self-confidence. It wasn't an acceptable, quiet kind of self-confidence. It was a brazen self-confidence, and they drew on it constantly, they lived off it. The surgeons were cool under pressure and they were helping people who really needed help. They took action, they took other people's brains into their own hands. There was suffering and pain, but there was work to be done and I got used to the endless cases of tumors and aneurysms and subdural hematomas. Every operation was an opportunity to relieve suffering and see something extraordinary: to see a brain, to see into a brain, a live brain, deep and pink with blood. Outside the OR, the hospitals were noisy and crowded. Outside the hospitals, the world was noisy and crowded and nobody was in charge. Inside the OR, it was a different story. One special thing brain surgeons know is what it really means to be the boss. Another thing they know is what it really means to make a mistake. For me, it all added up to a dynamic way to live. It was smart people doing very difficult things. It was long days full of rigor, risk, and reward. It hooked me.

A similar thing happened with my reading. As I worked my way through ever-more difficult books and learned more and more about the biochemistry and functional anatomy of the nervous system, I practically lost contact with the rest of the world. I buried myself in the material. Nothing was more interesting to me than whichever part of the nervous system I was studying or whichever incredible neurological phenomenon I was trying to understand. The hypothalamus, the blood-brain barrier, synaptic transmission, the nature of consciousness, the organization of the spinal cord, and on and on. The list is endless. All of it was new to me, all of it was a challenge, and all I wanted to do was read about it, talk about it, and think about it. And this wasn't simply a fascination with detail. I developed an absolute faith in biology. It was possible, I concluded, to understand the human nervous system and all of its functions as purely biological phenomena. It had to be so. The nervous system is an arrangement of cells—I'd written that sentence again and again—and all the answers to all the questions were there, in those cells. Had to be. Somehow. It was just a matter of time, time in the lab with the cells and time thinking. Not only would incurable neurological diseases eventually be cured, but the deeper mysteries of the human mind and life itself would be solved.

In each case I willingly and swiftly surrendered to a limited viewpoint because it offered a sense of order, a place to stand amidst the chaos and complexity of modern neurological medicine. That was a major part of both experiences. With a sense of order comes a sense of control, and in a place as potentially out of control as a major urban medical center, anything that enhances an individual's sense of control is to be valued, even if it means perpetuating a stereotype by becoming one.

Similarly, when one is confronted with something as daunting as the human nervous system, it is understandable to deal with it by reducing it to its parts. That is why, I believe, many young doctors and scientists automatically assume traditional roles and attitudes; not because they necessarily make for the best medicine or the best science, but because they are the fastest way to acquire that much-needed sense of control.

Of course a brain surgeon can't "operate" without assuming a certain level of power and exercising it. And a neuroscientist can't study the nervous system without breaking it down into its parts and believing in his science. Even as I reacted against my adopted perspectives, I recognized their necessity. Brain surgeons and neuroscientists, each in their own way, save lives and reduce pain and suffering. But as an outsider, I could see all too clearly the flip side. The difference between a confident surgeon who is very busy and an arrogant surgeon who doesn't have time for his patients is slim and critical, and it's a distinction that can easily be rendered moot for the patient. As for neuroscience, what I missed in most of what I read was a sense of the nervous system's wholeness and an acknowledgment of what I think of as its divine nature. It might seem naïve to point out that there is no listing for *soul* or *spirit* in the index of *Principles of Neural Science*, the field's most complete text, but that is exactly the problem.

What I realized, as a layman, was that the order and control I had found so appealing while working on this book were in fact functions of the distance that exists between doctor and patient, researcher and subject. For the doctor and patient, it's a cultural distance that originates in their wildly different kinds of knowledge and experience. The doctor knows *the body*, objectively and encyclopedically. The patient knows *a body*, his own, subjectively and instinctively. The distance between the two is increased and formalized by the hospital system, which, while ostensibly designed to meet the needs of the patient, as a matter of practice is organized around the needs of the doctor. With the neuroscientist and the nervous system, the distance is more conceptual. It stretches away in all directions from the shiny, overlit lab where the scientist wrestles with some specific, vital aspect of the thing to the dark, encompassing soul of the thing itself. Think of night in an enormous city of great buildings; all the windows are dark but one, and there a man is bent over a desk, concentrating, alone, while outside all around him yawns that deep living darkness. Suddenly he snaps his fingers and says, ''I've got it.'' Then he snaps off the lights. That's the kind of distance I'm talking about. So while the doctor's greater knowledge and experience quietly push him to keep his patients and their problems ''in perspective'' and at arm's length, the empirical demands of science require the scientist to study the human nervous system without ever approaching the messy metaphysical business of the human soul. And in the end, everybody gets off the hook, except of course the patients and the people who think life is more than just a matter of biology; they are left to sit and wonder what is going on.

This distance makes for modern medicine at its worst, which it is a lot of the time, and the clinical practice of neurological medicine at the end of the twentieth century is quintessentially modern. It is increasingly technological, specialized, and loaded with new and perplexing ethical questions about tissue transplants, life-support systems, genetic screening, and other complex issues. At the same time, ancient frustrations persist in the diseases that defy understanding and remain incurable. Today's young neurologists and neurosurgeons must absorb reams of new information their predecessors didn't have to worry about. And once they've performed the intellectual feat of mastering the material, they have to put it to work in an endless flow of patients, each of whom can justifiably demand the best treatment and fullest attention possible. In spite of a new emphasis in medical schools on compassion and the human side of medicine, it seems at times that there is little about modern medicine that doesn't militate against a positive personal experience for the patient and his doctor.

It's a complicated situation and it isn't going to get any simpler in the years ahead. Indeed, the one sure thing about the future is that there will be more of everything—more technology, more specialization, more patients, more bureaucracy, more knowledge, more moral and social issues. Ultimately, attitudes are going to make the difference, if there is to be a difference. The problem, however, is that daily experience shapes attitudes more than attitudes shape daily experience. A few weeks on the front lines in a busy hospital can turn the most well-meaning medical student into a disillusioned tough guy or, worse, a cynic. I've seen it happen and I think I understand it. What's needed is an attitude that can stand up to and transform the grinding daily experience, an attitude that can overcome the barriers that technology and specialization throw up between doctors and patients.

That's a powerful attitude, and not easy to come by. But it seems to me that it might grow out of a new, heightened appreciation of the natural wonder of the human nervous system. The idea is that every patient—good case, bad case, interesting case, boring case—embodies the very highest expression of nature. The ubiquitous human nervous system is the everyday, walking-around miracle, and every time a doctor comes into professional contact with it he is elevated. And I don't mean this as a flabby generalization. The way I see it, it works on the doctors' terms. That is, their technical, high-level knowledge of the nervous system positions them perfectly to make the necessary conceptual leap to a new attitude based on respect for the nervous system and the living spirit that arises in it and drives it. The root of the attitude is intellectual—neurosurgeons and neurologists understand the workings of the nervous system better than anybody and should be able to see it shining out at them at all times from the midst of everything else. They should not let all the routine crap come between them and this most extraordinary living thing. It is, after all, at the center of the medical system; it is the thing that all the great new machines are pointed at.

So instead of starting out with a head full of details

and a vague determination to be compassionate, an emotional impulse that clearly does not fare well in a modern hospital environment, the doctor simply acknowledges the obvious—that the human nervous systems deserves his best attention. Everything he knows about it reinforces that idea, and so does everything he doesn't know about it, which is a lot. Once that idea is in place, the next step is the logical one of recognizing the profound fact that the single greatest product of this single greatest natural entity is the individual human spirit. And now, with his feet planted solidly on an intellectual appreciation of the nervous system as a medical marvel, the doctor can reach for the emotional fruit I believe this approach will bear. Because the point is that the pain-in-the-ass meningioma in Room 605 is special precisely because he is a pain-in-the-ass and not at all like his quiet roommate, the aneurysm. The same goes for the junkie with a concussion in the ER at 4:00 A.M. and the recidivist phantom backache at Thursday's clinic. They are all exceptional individuals with nervous systems beyond any doctor's complete comprehension. But if the pressures of modern medicine make it so difficult for the doctors to relate to them as who they are, then let them start by relating to them as what they are. It's an approach that is consistent with the facts of modern medical life because an intellectual approach to the nervous system, scrupulously pursued, eventually leads to the emotional reality of a single human being. Because the what of us is the who of us, and they are inseparable. The payoff: a genuine, resilient kind of compassion that emerges as the doctor proves to himself that each of his many patients is in fact one of a kind, unique and alone among men.

For the neuroscientist, the idea is the same. A cellular approach to the functions of the nervous system is logical and effective; and human behavior is, to a large extent, a matter of biology. But any attempt to understand human behavior that doesn't take into account the spiritual element of human life is incomplete, a failure of imagination. Even if it is possible to delineate the exact structures, chemicals, and steps involved in the generation of a specific emotion, and someone does it, that won't mean they will have localized the emotion itself. Yes, love is a chemical reaction, but there is more to it than that. There is, I believe, something beyond biology, and it is a factor, somehow, in the function of every living human cell and in every human thought and deed. In a sense, the human nervous system is a complex set of conditions necessary for the existence of the soul. But that is wrong in that it implies a separateness, and there is none. Ultimately, all research into the workings of the nervous system leads to the soul, and all neuroscientists are working in its shadow. Acknowledging the shadow would transform it into a great light, and the work would shine with a new significance, hard science informed by an awareness of the holy unknown.

In the end, I guess, it's a matter of faith. If the future is to be worth the trouble of getting there, that is what it will take—faith in man, faith in the human nervous system, faith in its power, its perfection, and its instinctive, insatiable need to understand itself.

SELECTED BIBLIOGRAPHY

Adams, R. D., and Victor, M. *Principles of Neurology*. McGraw-Hill, 1977, 1981.

Blakemore, C. *Mechanics of the Mind*. Cambridge University Press, 1977.

The Brain. A Scientific American Book. W. H. Freeman, 1979.

The Brain and Its Functions: A Symposium. Charles C. Thomas, 1958.

Calvin, W. H., and Ojemann, G. A. *Inside the Brain*. New American Library, 1980.

Caroscio, J. T., ed. *Amyotrophic Lateral Sclerosis: A Guide For Patient Care*. Thieme, 1986.

Castiglioni, A. *A History of Medicine*. Knopf, 1947.

Duquesne, T., and Reeves, J. *A Handbook of Psychoactive Medicines*. Quartet Books, 1982.

Freeman, W., and Watts, J. W. *Psychosurgery in the Treatment of Mental Disorders and Intractable Pain*. Charles C. Thomas, 1950.

Fulton, J. *Harvey Cushing: A Biography*. Knopf, 1946.

Gunther, J. *Death Be Not Proud*. Harper & Row, 1949.

Kandel, E. R., and Schwartz, J. *Principles of Neural Science*. Elsevier, 1985.

Luria, A. R. *The Working Brain: An Introduction to Neuropsychology*. Basic Books, 1973.

Mettler, C. C. *History of Medicine*, edited by F. A. Mettler. Blakiston, 1947.

McHenry, L. C., Jr. *Garrison's History of Neurology*. Charles C. Thomas, 1969.

Muldur, D. W., ed. *The Diagnosis and Treatment of Amyotrophic Lateral Sclerosis*. Houghton Mifflin, 1980.

Noback, C. R., and Demarest, R. J. *The Nervous System: Introduction and Review*. McGraw-Hill, 1986, 1977, 1972.

Nolte, J. *The Human Brain: An Introduction to Its Functional
Anatomy*. C. V. Mosby, 1981.

Penfield, W., and Roberts, L. *Speech and Brain-Mechanisms*.
Princeton University Press, 1959.

Pincus, J. H., and Tucker, G. J. *Behavioral Neurology*. Oxford
University Press, 1985.

Restak, R. M. *The Brain*. Bantam, 1984.

Restak, R. M. *The Brain: The Last Frontier*. Doubleday, 1979.

Riese, W. *A History of Neurology*. MD Books, 1959.

Walker, A. E., ed. *A History of Neurological Surgery*. Hafner,
1967, 1951.

Sarno, M. T., ed. *Acquired Aphasia*. Academic Press, 1981.

Spillane, J. D. *The Doctrine of the Nerves*. Oxford University
Press, 1981.

ACKNOWLEDGMENTS

This book is based on my firsthand observations of the clinical practice of neurology and neurosurgery, and extensive interviews with doctors, patients, researchers, and others involved in the world of neurological medicine.

The people I acknowledge here, the people who made this book possible, let me into a very private, intimate world. They opened up to me and gave me straight answers. They helped me to see what was happening and to understand what I was seeing. They also did the extra thing, and left me alone to write my book and draw my own conclusions. I thank them for their honesty, their enthusiasm, and their trust.

At the Neurological Institute of New York, Bennett M. Stein was cooperative from the very beginning. His operating room was the first one I entered, and he gave me the start I needed to get this project going and to keep it going. His counterpart in the department of neurology, Lewis P. Rowland, introduced me to the mysteries of his speciality, and his interest in my work was an inspiration and a challenge. It was at Neuro that I first met Phillip Cogen, who was then a chief resident. His involvement throughout the long course of this project has been invaluable. In addition, the following neurosurgeons and neurologists let me watch them at work and many of them sat for interviews during my two tours of duty at Neuro: John L. Antunes, Henry Brem, John C. M. Brust, Jr., Robert E. Burke, Peter W. Carmel, Duncan B. Carpenter, Lisa DeAngelis, Darryl C. Devivo, Paul W. Diefenback, Matthew E. Fink, Linda R.

Kaplan, Alan D. Legatt, Christopher M. Loftus, Kenneth M. Louis, Richard Mayeux, Jost W. Michelsen, Jay P. Mohr, Kalman D. Post, Donald O. Quest, Saran S. Rosner, Mitchell J. Rubin, Todd C. Sacktor, Robert A. Solomon, Abe Steinberger, David S. Younger, and Steven J. Zuckerman. Also, J. Lawrence Pool, professor emeritus of neurological surgery, whose thirty-six years at Neuro included twenty-three as head of the neurosurgery department, gave me an interview.

At Stanford University Medical Center, I gratefully acknowledge the cooperation of John W. Hanbery, the head of the department of neurosurgery, as well as Frances Conley, Lawrence Shuer, and Gary Steinberg.

At the Rusk Institute, Martha Taylor Sarno and her staff showed me what it takes to confront aphasia.

At UCLA, Keith Nuechterlein and Arnold Scheibel helped me learn to think about thought in a new way.

At UC-Irvine, Monte S. Buchsbaum and his colleagues enabled me to look into working brains, and into the future.

Lynn Klein and her associates at the ALS Association were a key source of information about that terrible disease.

Special thanks go to Gail Belsky.

Most of all, I want to thank the many patients I met in the course of my research. They were the most dynamic element in the dynamic world of neurological medicine, and their courage amazed me time and again. Lance Meagher is the only one in the book whose name has not been changed and whose identifying details have not been altered. Others appear in disguise to protect their privacy and still others do not appear at all. But every patient I met is in this book, somehow, because every one I met is in my heart.

Others who deserve thanks, now that this journey is done, include my sprawling family, my friends, and my many colleagues in the journalism trade. My agent, Esther Newberg, kept the faith and hung in with me to the end. My editor, Alice Mayhew, believed in this book from the start, and kept me at the task with regular doses of insight. Working to her standards was the greatest challenge of my professional life. David Shipley solved problems large and small, and worked hard to turn my manuscript into a book. George Hodgman contributed his good ideas at just the right moment.

Finally, I want to acknowledge two people who played important roles in my life as a writer: Ruth Cochrane, a teacher who was also a friend; and the late Jaakov Kohn, a friend who was also a teacher.

INDEX

About the Author

DAVID NOONAN'S writing has appeared in *Esquire*, *The New York Times Magazine*, *Sports Illustrated*, and other publications. He lives in Los Angeles, California, with his wife and son, and is currently at work on a novel.

again I sight the instrument to